Mindfulness
THE MASTER KEY

Mindfulness
THE MASTER KEY

SWAMI CHAITANYA KEERTI

wisdom
tree

© Author

First published 2016

ISBN 978-81-8328-459-2

Published by
Wisdom Tree
4779/23, Ansari Road
Darya Ganj, New Delhi-110 002
Ph.: 011-23247966/67/68
wisdomtreebooks@gmail.com

Printed in India

Contents

Self in Silence

Introduction

I dive down into the depth of the ocean of forms,
hoping to gain the perfect pearl of the formless.

—Rabindranath Tagore

This collection of Swami Chaitanya Keerti's columns, written over a period of time, indicates the intensity of his spiritual search, as well as the depth of his understanding. As Tagore says in the lines from *Gitanjali* quoted above, the aspirant dives into the deep sea, much like a diver in search of a pearl that is as rare as it is elusive. When he dives in, there is no guarantee that he will find anything other than empty shells. The process is arduous and often filled with doubt and self-conflict. The fact that the aspirant does emerge with a 'perfect pearl'—of enlightenment, insight, awakening—can only be described as a miracle.

For Swamiji, the ocean he dives in time and time again is undoubtedly the wisdom of his Master, Osho. For many of us, it is difficult to fathom the entire breadth of Osho's teachings, so wide and varied are they in their spiritual and intellectual reach. Upon reading Osho's extensive commentaries on texts as complex as the *Vijnana Bhairava Tantra* and as obscure as *The Book of Mirdad,* and his expositions of the teachings of legendary teachers like the Buddha,

Jesus, Kabir and Lao Tzu among others, one can only marvel at the truly 'oceanic' nature of Osho's wisdom. Osho is the kind of guru who is not just an illuminator of ignorance; his luminescence is as close to being an actual source of spiritual light as can be hoped for in human incarnation.

Swami Chaitanya Keerti, who has had the good fortune of directly receiving the Master's teachings, emerges not just as an ideal conveyor of these teachings, but one who is able to tailor them according to this day and age, as the need might be. This happens several times in the book, as in the chapter, 'Meditation: An Individual Revolution', where he comments on a cover story in *Time* magazine on the 'mindfulness revolution' sweeping the US, and places mindfulness in its proper meditative context. Or in 'The Escape Within', where he tackles the trauma caused by earthquakes with a Zen story that exhorts one to go within when there is an upheaval without.

It appears that Swamiji has been able to absorb the Master's wisdom, arrived at a place of knowing regarding the truth that they point to, and put them into actual practice in the world. In this sense, he is able to not just look at the 'finger that points to the moon', as the Master would be described in Zen terms, but actually see and experience the moon of spiritual wisdom for himself. Swamiji's words, in that sense, act as pointers to others, those of us struggling on the spiritual path.

So closely intertwined are his words with his Master's, separated only by quotation marks, that both teacher and disciple appear to inhabit the same continuum of consciousness. While the disciple's understanding is of course derived from the teacher's, it is not derivative in an ordinary sense of the word. It is important to understand this difference, for Swami Chaitanya Keerti quotes Osho a lot, and often seems to be revisiting the Master's words. But the freshness of perspective is all his own, while the derivation is a spiritual and inspirational one, and should not be confused with or mistaken for intellectual slavishness.

One endearing quality of Osho's teachings, which Swami Chaitanya Keerti seems to have imbibed from his Master, is that of witty repartee, coupled with the rendering of weighty philosophy in easy-to-understand everyday language. Anecdotes and jokes are employed to dispel the reader's mental lethargy and freshen the mind to keep it alert to the task at hand of understanding that which is being said.

For readers interested in spirituality, this book has the potential of becoming a credible and trustworthy companion on the path. For those who are looking for something deeper in their lives but do not quite know what it is, this book can be a starting point, the beginning of an adventure that is sure to last at least one lifetime, if not many.

—Swati Chopra

MASTER

OF YOUR

BEING

Mindfulness: An Individual Revolution

'Few of us ever live in the present. We are forever anticipating what is to come or remembering what has gone,' said Louis L'Amour, the bestselling author of *The Lonesome Gods* and other works of fiction. It's possible he may have read some of Osho's books while Osho was in the United States.

Meditation, living each moment with total awareness, in a relaxed way, has always been the central message of Osho's discourses. Such insights of mindfulness have touched the hearts of many creative people around the world. This is indeed a modern term for meditation that has been known to spiritual seekers since the time of Gautama Buddha, who practised and taught Vipassana and *Anapansatiyoga*. It might have been there even before him since the time of the Upanishads and Lord Shiva. But what can be said very conclusively is that Gautama Buddha was the first spiritual scientist who articulated it in such a way that the modern scientific world, without any blind faith, understands it and does research on it also. *Time* magazine has published a cover story on this subject. It was titled: 'The Mindful Revolution'.

Gautama Buddha is reported to have said in one of his *gathas*:

'Once a man came unto me and denounced me on account of my observing the way and practising great loving kindness. But I kept silent and did not answer him. The denunciation ceased. I then asked him, "If you bring a present to your neighbour and he accepts it not, does the present come back to you?" The man replied, "It will." I said, "You denounce me now but as I accept it not, you must take the wrong deed back upon your own person." It is like an echo succeeding sound, it is like shadow following object. You never escape the effect of your own evil deeds. Be therefore mindful and cease from doing evil.'

One stops doing any evil when one is mindful, in a state of meditation, each moment. In such a state we do not react, we simply respond meditatively. Reaction is most of the time very mechanical and automatic. Response takes place when there is relaxed awareness, a watchfulness, a passive alertness. Response is from a state of consciousness which is rooted in freedom. Reaction is born out of tension and leading to more tension. It creates entanglement, chain of actions and bondage. Mindfulness means being responsive to every situation in life, each moment with total awareness.

Osho elaborates: 'So whenever there is a need to respond, the first thing is become mindful, become aware. Remember your centre. Become grounded in your centre. Be there for a few moments before you do anything. There is no need to think about it because thinking is partial. There is no need to feel about it because feeling is partial. There is no need to find clues from your parents, Bible, Koran, Gita...there is no need. You simply remain tranquil, silent, simply alert—watching the situation as if you are absolutely out of it, aloof, a watcher on the hills. This is the first requirement—to be centred whenever you want to act. Then out of this centring let the act arise and whatsoever you do will be virtuous, whatsoever you do will be right. Buddha said, "Right mindfulness is the only virtue there is. Not to be mindful is to fall into error. To act unconsciously is to fall into error."'

To conclude, let us recall one of the quotes of Louis L'Amour who wrote in one of his books: 'Long since, I had learned that one needs moments of quiet, moments of stillness, for both the inner and outer man, a moment of contemplation or even simple emptiness when the stress could ease away and a calmness enter the tissues. Such moments of quiet gave one strength, gave one coolness of mind with which to approach the world and its problems sometimes but a few minutes were needed.'

Just Be Yourself in Your Prayerfulness

There's a very beautiful story about a Hassid mystic, Zusia. Osho considers him as one of the most beautiful mystics this world has known. He was a man of prayer and a very sensitive human being.

It is said that once he was going into the hills and he saw many birds, caught by a man, in a cage. Zusia opened the cage—because birds are meant to fly—and all the birds flew away.

The man who had encaged the birds came rushing out of his house and said, 'What have you done?'

And Zusia said 'Birds are meant to fly. Look how beautiful they look on the wing!'

But the man thought otherwise and became infuriated. His whole day's work had been destroyed as he had been hoping to go to the market and sell the birds and there were many, many things to be done—and now Zusia had ruined the whole thing.

He gave Zusia a good beating. This did not provoke any anger in Zusia. He kept laughing as if he was enjoying being beaten. The man thought Zusia must be a mad man. After a while, Zusia asked the man, 'Are you done with the beating or would you like to do a little more? Are you finished? Please tell because now I have to go.' The man could not answer. What could he answer? This man was simply mad! And Zusia started singing a song. He was very happy—happy that the birds were flying in the sky and happy that he was beaten and yet, it didn't hurt, happy that he could receive it as a gift, happy that he could still thank God. There was no complaint. This way Zusia transformed the whole quality of the situation.

Zusia always knew how to transform anger into compassion. He had a very unique way of praying. At the time of his death, when he was praying, tears were flowing down from his eyes and he was trembling.

Somebody asked him, 'What is the matter? Why are you trembling?'

He said, 'I am trembling for a certain reason. This is my last moment, I am dying. Soon I will be facing my God and I am certain he is not going to ask me "Zusia, why were you not a Moses?"

If he asks, I will say, "Lord, because you didn't give me the qualities of a Moses!" and there will be no problem. He will not ask me "Why were you not the Rabbi Akiba?" But if he asks, I will tell him, "Sir, you never gave me the qualities of being an Akiba, that's why." But I am trembling because if he asks "Zusia, why were you not a Zusia?" then I will have nothing to answer, then I will have to look down in shame. That's why I am trembling and these tears are flowing. My whole life, I tried to become Moses or Akiba or somebody else and I completely forgot that he wanted me to be just Zusia and nobody else. Now I am trembling, now I am afraid. If he asks this question, what am I going to answer? How will I be able to raise my eyes when he says "Why were you not Zusia? You were given all the qualities of being a Zusia, how did you miss?" And I have missed being myself in imitating others.'

This kind of humbleness is really unique.

Mind is the Jailer

'There is something beyond our mind which abides in silence. It is the supreme mystery beyond thought. Let your mind and subtle body rest upon that and not on anything else.' It is important to remember these beautiful words of the *Maitri Upanishad*, when the world is filled with hatred and noisy slugfest.

What is beyond our mind, which abides in silence? It is our consciousness. It is our heart. And being totally intoxicated by our mind and its manipulations, we tend to forget who we truly are. Our consciousness feeds on peace and our heart expands with love, but our mind, when it monopolises our whole being, makes our life a battlefield. This is the downhill path of misery. It shrinks our vision and narrows it to make it a tunnel vision. We become totally selfish and violent, thinking of others as our enemies. This is a very unnatural state of being. The consciousness wants to fly high in the open sky and the heart yearns for love but the mind is always preoccupied with animosity towards others. The mind creates Pandavas and Kauravas—the holy and the unholy. The consciousness knows that God's creation is all divine—it is *Vasudhaiva Kutumbakam*, one family of universal brotherhood. All divisions are fictitious and illusory. This is the *mayajaal* of the mind. When our consciousness transcends the divisions created by our mind, we feel others not as others but as ourselves. We transcend the artificial confinements.

Osho reminds us: 'When one remembers one's sacredness, one's infinity, joy wells up. When one thinks of oneself as limited by a thousand and one limitations, misery arises because a limitation is a kind of confinement; it is a prison. How can one be happy in such a small body? How can one be happy in such a petty mind? It is impossible. They don't allow you space to dance, to sing, to celebrate. One is cluttered, one is like a junkyard. One needs the vast sky. In that vastness is freedom. In that freedom is joy.

'Fall in love with the transcendental...search for it. And I call it "falling in love" because the search has to be through the heart and not through the mind. If you search through the mind, you will never go beyond the mind. The mind is very jealous and it won't allow you to surpass it; it is very possessive. The mind is the jailer, it guards the gate. It won't allow you to go beyond the limits. You can function within the limits—it gives you all freedom within the limits—but don't step outside; that is not allowed. The heart is not a prison, it is an opening; it is a door, not a wall. Hence, I say "fall in love with the beyond".'

Friedrich Nietzsche said, 'That day will be the most unfortunate when man stops surpassing himself.' When the arrow of human consciousness does not have anything like a target beyond itself, that day will be the most unfortunate. But that day will never come, it cannot come—the urge is built-in. Man is man only because of the desire to surpass himself...that very desire is his humanness. Our mind finds fault with everything and everybody. But if we see meditatively, with the pure vision of consciousness, everything looks perfect and beautiful. You just approach this great shrine of God. God is enshrined here in every stone, and every stone is a sermon, and He is flowering in every flower, and He is breathing in every heart. You just approach with innocence.

Find a Purpose

Patrick Hill, a researcher at Carleton University in Canada, has published a very significant study in the journal *Psychological Science*. His finding points out that a sense of purpose in life and setting overarching goals to achieve that target may help us live longer, no matter what our age. He concludes that the earlier someone finds a direction for their life, the earlier its protective effects begin.

There is a beautiful story of Rohini from the days of Gautama Buddha which proves this fact. On one occasion, Buddha's disciple Anuruddha visited Kapilavastu. While he was staying at the monastery there, all his relatives, with the exception of his sister Rohini, came to see him. On learning from them that Rohini had not come because she was suffering from leprosy, he sent for her. Rohini came to see her brother but covered her head in shame. Feeling very sorry for his sister, Anuruddha advised her to do some meritorious deeds. He suggested that she should sell some of her jewellery and with the money gained, build a refectory for bhikkhus.

Rohini agreed to do as she was told. Anuruddha also asked his other relatives to help in the construction of the hall. Further, he told Rohini to sweep the floor and fill the water pots every day, even while the construction was on. She did as instructed and began to get better. This inspired her to put her whole energy into this noble work. A miracle happened and 90 per cent of her leprosy disappeared during this period when she was totally involved in this work. She was visualising bhikkhus meditating in the hall in the presence of the Buddha, their faces glowing with divine energy and she sitting in satsang with them. This visualisation transformed Rohini's whole being.

When the construction of the hall was completed, the Buddha and his bhikkhus were invited to have food, which had been donated as alms. After the meal, the Buddha asked for the donor of the building and the alms but Rohini was not there. The Buddha sent for her. When she came, he asked her whether she knew why she had been inflicted with the dreaded disease. She did not. Buddha told her that she had done an evil deed in one of her past lives. Rohini was, at one time, the chief queen of the king of Varanasi. It so happened that the king had a favourite dancer and Rohini was very jealous of her. The queen wanted to punish the dancer. Thus, one day, she had her attendants put some itching powder made from cowage pods in the dancer's bed, her blankets, etc.

Next, they called the dancer and as though in jest, threw some itching powder on her. The girl started itching all over and ran to her room and bed, which made her suffer even more. As a result of that evil deed, Rohini had become a leper in her existing life. The Buddha then exhorted the congregation not to act foolishly in anger and not to bear any ill will towards others.

Then the Buddha gave the following sutra to his bhikkhus: 'Give up anger, abandon conceit, overcome all fetters. Ills of life (*dukkha*) do not befall one who does not cling to mind and body and is free from moral defilements.'

At that moment, Rohini also attained total freedom—her skin disease disappeared and her complexion became fair, smooth and glowed with good health.

You are Invincible!

We live in an ever-changing world. But there are very few people who understand this change as the nature of the world and flow with it. Most of us try to swim upstream and turn life into a struggle. Those who know that change is inevitable also know that change always occurs on the outside, while within it is a never-changing centre.

The art of meditation is to find a centre within one's being. Just an hour of such relaxation can rejuvenate and unleash immense creativity in us. Those who meditate know this secret.

Osho tells us: 'Please be re-established in your centre, be aware of the centre, which is unmoving and allow the whole existence to move. It's not a disturbance at all. It becomes a disturbance only if you cling to it. Then you are falling into absurdities, foolish efforts. They will not succeed—you will be a failure.... Know well that life changes but somewhere within this change, there is also an unmoving centre. Just become aware of it. That awareness is enough to liberate you. That very feeling that "I am unmoving" liberates. That is the truth!'

Osho talks about a significant incident in the life of Alexander the Great who was returning to Macedon from India. Friends requested him to bring an Indian sannyasi with him. They said,

'When you come with conquered possessions, don't forget to bring home a sannyasi. What type of a man renounces the world?'

And so, Alexander asked his soldiers to go in search of a sannyasi. The soldiers asked an old man who said, 'Yes, yes, there is a great sannyasi. But it will be difficult to persuade him to go to Macedon with Alexander.'

The soldiers retorted, 'Don't you worry about that. We can force anyone. Just tell us where he is.'

So, the soldiers reached Dandami, a sannyasi who was standing naked at the riverbank and said, 'Alexander orders you to come with us. Every care will be taken, there will be no inconvenience, you will be a royal guest. But you have to come with us to Athens.'

The sannyasi laughed and said, 'No force in this world can force me to follow. You won't understand, so it's better that you bring Alexander to me.' Hearing this, Alexander felt insulted but still wanted to see the sage. He came with a sword and roared, 'If you say no, then you'll lose your life. I will cut off your head.'

The sannyasi again laughed and said, 'You're a little late. You cannot kill me now because I have killed myself already. You can cut off my head but you cannot cut me. So when this head falls down on earth, you will see it falling down and I will also see it falling down. But you cannot cut me; you cannot even touch me. So don't waste time...you can cut! Raise your sword and cut off my head.'

Alexander the Great couldn't kill that man. It was impossible because it was useless. The man was so beyond death, it was impossible to kill him. You can only be killed if you cling to life. That clinging to the changing pattern makes you a mortal.

If you do not cling, you are as you have always been—immortal. Immortality is your birthright, it has always been there. So there is no need to force the changing periphery to be static. It will go on. All that you need to know is that you aren't the wheel. You are only the axis!

When You're Angry and You Know It...

With such cut-throat competition, hate and greed around us, it is tough to stay happy. Getting negative vibes and feeling jealous is a normal state of mind for many of us. But there is a technique by which you can counter this life condition. If you get angry with someone, do not project that mood on that person—stay centred.

Osho explains: 'If hate arises for someone or against someone or love arises for someone, what do we do? We project it on to the person. If you hate me, you are bound to forget yourself in your hate, only I become your object. If you love me, you forget yourself completely; only I become the object. You project your love or hate or whatsoever you feel upon me. You completely forget the inner centre of your own being; the other becomes your centre.'

'I love you' is the most common manifestation of the feeling that you are the source of my love. But it is not really so. I am the source; you are just a screen onto which I project my love. And I feel that you are the source! This is not fact, this is fiction. I draw my love and project it onto you. In that love-energy projected onto you, you become lovely. You may not be lovely to someone else.

You may be absolutely repulsive to someone else. Why? Because we are just projecting our moods onto others.

So when you are in a foul mood, remember that you are the source. So do not move to the other, move to the source. When you feel hatred, do not go to the object. Go to the nucleus. Do not go to the person from whom it is coming but to your own centre. Look within! Use your hate, love or anger as a journey to move towards your inner centre. Move to the source and try to stay centred.

Try it…it is a scientific and psychological technique. When someone insults you, there is a sudden burst of anger towards the person who has insulted you and you will project this anger onto him. But he has not done anything. If he has insulted you, what has he done? He has just pricked you and drawn out the anger from your life. But what you need to understand is that the anger is yours and yours alone!

If you throw a bucket into a dry well, nothing will come out. But if you throw a bucket into a well full of water, a bucket full of water will come out. But the water is from the well and the bucket only helps to bring it out.

So, a person who insults you is just throwing a bucket onto you. And that's how a bucket full of anger, hate or vengeance that is within you will come out. You are the source. Challenge yourself to change that!

There is a very mysterious Tao sutra: How does the true man of Tao walk through walls without obstruction and stand in fire without being burnt?

Osho explains this with his unique vision: 'Someone asked Chuang Tzu, "We have heard that a man of Tao can walk through walls without obstruction. How?" If you don't have any obstruction within you, no obstruction can obstruct you. This is the rule. If you have no resistance within you, in your heart, the whole world is open for you. There is no resistance. The world is just a reflection, it is a big mirror; if you have resistance then the whole world has resistance.'

This is very difficult for the ego to understand. Ego is the wall within us and ego is the main resistance. Ego is in conflict with others and others are also not without ego. This is the reason that the world is full of violence. And a violent man is violent not only towards others, he is also violent towards nature. This is the basic cause of destruction of nature.

Osho says: 'Fight will give you a stronger ego. It will shape you. So fight the mother, fight the father, fight the teacher, fight the society. Life is struggle. And Darwin started the whole trend when he said only the fittest survive; life means survival of the fittest. So the stronger you are in your ego, the more chance you will have of surviving. The West lives through politics, the East has a totally different attitude...and Tao is the core, the very essence of the Eastern consciousness. It says: No individuality, no ego, no fight, become one with the mother; there is no enemy, the question is not of conquering. Even a man, a very knowledgeable man, a very penetrating, logical man like Bertrand Russell, thinks in terms of conquest—conquering nature. Science seems to be a struggle, a fight with nature: How to break the lock, how to open the secrets, how to grab the secrets from nature.

'Eastern consciousness is totally different. Eastern consciousness says: Ego is the problem, do not make it stronger, do not create any fight. And not the fittest but the humblest survive. That is why I insist again and again that Jesus is from the East; that is why he could not be understood in the West. The West has misunderstood him. The East could have understood him because the East knows Lao Tzu, Chuang Tzu, Buddha, and Jesus belongs to them. He says: "Those who are last will be the first in my kingdom of God. The humblest, the meekest will possess the kingdom of God." The poor in spirit is the goal. Who is poor in spirit? The empty boat, he who is not at all—no claim on anything, no possession of anything, no self. He lives as an absence.

'Nature gives her secrets. There is no need to grab, there is no need to kill, there is no need to break the lock. Love nature, and nature gives you her secrets. Love is the key. Conquering is absurd. So what has happened in the West? This conquering has destroyed the whole of nature. So, now there is a cry for ecology, how to restore the balance. We have destroyed nature completely because we have broken all the locks and we have destroyed the whole balance. And now through that imbalance, humanity will die sooner or later.'

It seems that we have come to a point where nothing can be done—it is very hopeless. So we do nothing. What we actually do is that we do not feel responsible ourselves and continue to blame it on others. This has to stop if we want the balance of nature to be restored. The first thing is to realise this and then have an intention, feel strongly about it. With this spirit in our heart, we should bring clarity in our vision. Meditation will give us this vision.

Osho reminds and warns us: 'The world is being poisoned very slowly. The rivers are being polluted, the oceans are being polluted, the lakes are dying. Nature is being destroyed. We are exploiting the earth so much that sooner or later we will not be able to live on it. We are not behaving well with nature. Our whole approach is wrong, it is destructive. We only take from the earth and we never give anything back. We only exploit nature. The ecology is broken, the circulation is broken; we are not living in a perfect circle and nature is a perfect circle: If you take from one hand and you give from another, you do not destroy it. But we are doing it. We only go on taking and all the resources are being spent. But this poisoning is happening slowly. You do not see it happening because it takes a long time. And then there are politicians who go on gathering more and more atomic weapons—more atom bombs, more hydrogen bombs as if man has decided to commit suicide.'

Loneliness: The Personal Demon

I have heard that in the beginning of the world, God was feeling very lonely, as he had no fun in his life. Just being and being could not be interesting even to God. So, he thought of getting into some creativity and doing something—and the first thing he did was to create Adam in his own image. God was self-congratulatory and admired his own creativity. He kept an eye on Adam for a few days to find out how his creation was. One day, he asked Adam: 'Howdy doody? How do you do, my son?'

Adam replied: 'I am feeling bored and lonely. I need some fun in my life. It would be nice to have a companion.'

God meditated for a moment and told Adam: 'So be it! Soon you will have a very interesting companion.'

Out of the blue, God created Eve who was an interesting companion indeed. Adam was overjoyed. This joy remained for a few days and then again Adam started feeling miserable. Adam was not lonely but somewhat uncomfortable and bored again. He complained to God. God, expressing his helplessness, told him: 'My son, you asked for it, now you deal with it. Be intelligent.'

Since then Adam has been trying to be intelligent and dealing with this strange situation. The more he tries to solve anything, the more it gets complicated. He suffers being together with Eve as much as he suffered without her.

From ancient Adam to modern hero Leonardo DiCaprio, this double dilemma of loneliness and being together continues to torment human beings. Recently, Leonardo DiCaprio told the media that being alone was his 'personal demon'. The forty-one-year-old actor admits he struggles to cope when he is not surrounded by his friends and family and suffered from depression when he shot the movie *Shutter Island*.

He said: 'The loneliness is my personal demon. During the shooting of the movie it was like I fell into a black hole and was totally depressed.

'You're cut off from friends, family and your girlfriend. That's brutal. The world kept turning while I was stuck on the set. It's like a strange form of everyday amnesia.'

This is the price of being rich and famous that people like Leonardo DiCaprio pay for their achievements. The poor have to struggle a lot and stay away from their family to earn money. And the rich become so busy in their ambitious projects that they cannot find quality time to be with their family or friends. That is why everybody is feeling so miserable in the world. *Nanak Dukhiya Sab Sansar*. Guru Nanak observes that the whole world is miserable. Gautama Buddha says the same. Anybody can see that the world we have created for ourselves is full of misery.

What is the way out? The way out is the way in—as suggested by the enlightened ones. Meditate and find happiness in your heart.

Osho says: 'First, become alone. First, start enjoying yourself. First, love yourself. First, become so authentically happy that if nobody comes it doesn't matter; you are full, overflowing. If nobody knocks at your door, it is perfectly okay—you are not missing. You are not waiting for somebody to come and knock at the door. You are at home. If somebody comes, good, beautiful. If nobody comes that too is beautiful and good.

'Then move into relationship. Now you move like a master, not like a beggar. Now you move like an emperor, not like a beggar. And the person who has lived in his aloneness will always be attracted to another person who is also living in his aloneness beautifully because the same attracts the same. When two masters meet—masters of their being, of their aloneness—happiness is not just added, it is multiplied. It becomes a tremendous phenomenon of celebration. And they don't exploit, they share. They don't use each other. Rather, on the contrary, they both become one and enjoy the existence that surrounds them.'

SINGING

ONE'S

SONG

Fragrance of Love

Once a disciple told his master, 'Every day you give profound discourses that transform lives. Wouldn't it be nice if we compile these into books and preserve them for the future generations? These books will preserve your name for eternity and the money could be utilised to build an ashram and meet our daily expenses.'

The master replied: 'Yes, it is a good idea to publish them. But remember that the profoundness and the force that you feel in my discourses are not mine—it is the Divine that is speaking through me. I don't own these discourses. I am just like a hollow bamboo and the divine song is flowing through me. When a mystic creates, he is only a medium, a hollow bamboo on the lips of God, which becomes a flute.

'The flute of the infinite is played without ceasing, and its sound is love: When love renounces all limits, it reaches truth. How widely the fragrance spreads! The song is His; the flute cannot sing, the flute can only allow the singing to flow through. Existence is a passage; so is man. Man is a flute. So are the birds, trees, the sun and the moon.'

The profound messages that were given by Krishna, Buddha, Jesus, Mohammad, Nanak, Kabir, Meera and the unknown ancient sages of the Upanishads are divine in the ultimate sense.

The Upanishads contain the purest message and the most interesting thing is that we don't know the authors. The enlightened ones do not share their teachings for any worldly gain, name or fame. If they did, their teachings become very mundane. The truth flows through them and they do not compromise with those who have any vested interest to distort their truth. They take the risk of being misunderstood and be harassed but they never compromise. Jesus was crucified for the sake of truth. The truth does not belong to a person—it is divine and universal.

The disciple had another question: 'Beloved Master, there are some fake gurus who are stealing your words and are preaching to the masses. Shall we copyright your words to protect them so that nobody can steal them?'

The master responded: 'The truth is not mine. The words are not mine. I do not own the truth and the words. The same has always been expressed by the awakened ones and the same will always be expressed in the future. So do not bother to copyright truth and the words. Do not do such things to embarrass me. If you really want to do something, then share this unconditionally. I tell you the same what Jesus said to his disciples, "Go to the rooftops and shout the truth from there because people are deaf. Unless you shout they are not going to hear." It should reach far and wide without any restrictions and barriers. No need to limit. No need to control. The flower of enlightenment has bloomed, let the fragrance ride on the breeze and touch the hearts. Do not create any hindrances.'

The disciple agreed then but when his master left his body, he forgot all of these and went ahead to copyright the words of his master. Osho says: 'Things can be copyrighted, thoughts cannot be copyrighted and certainly meditations cannot be copyrighted. They are not things of the marketplace. Nobody can monopolise anything. But perhaps the West cannot understand the difference between an objective commodity and an inner experience. For ten thousand years, the East has been meditating and nobody has put trademarks upon meditations.'

The Knot of Love

There are friends and there are enemies—and there are brothers, sisters and other relations. We see them loving each other and there are moments when they are ready to die for each other and then, there are moments when they are full of hate for each other—so much so that they can kill each other.

Strangely, the same people who were once in love, now hate and want to kill each other. The sudden change from love to hate and in rare cases, from hate to love, makes us wonder how and why this happens. It happens between husbands and wives, girlfriends and boyfriends, brothers and sisters, and other such relationships.

There is always a conflict in relationships. And this conflict starts developing very early in childhood when children observe that they are not getting enough love or attention from parents, while their younger/elder brother or sister is getting all the love and attention. Such situations can create an inferiority complex or self-pity in children and they can become violent. The same can happen in school and classrooms also.

This is a very unhealthy and toxic beginning of life for kids. According to Dr Albert Adler, a famous psychologist, 'Kid squabbling is really based on subconscious striving for power.'

Osho says, 'The mother may love one child more, another a

little less. You cannot expect that she should love absolutely equally; it is not possible. Children are very perceptive. They can immediately see that somebody is liked more and somebody is liked less. They know that this pretension of the mother's loving them equally is just bogus. So an inner conflict, fight and ambition arises.'

Children are simple and simple things work for them. Osho says: 'Don't say to the child, "Love me because I am your mother." It may create incapacity in the child, and he will not be able to love anyone else. Then it happens that grown-up children—I call them grown-up children—continue to be fixed. So you cannot love your wife because deep inside you can love only your mother. But your wife is not your mother and your mother cannot be your wife, so you continue to be fixed—a mother fixation.... You go on expecting things from your wife as if she is your mother—not consciously. If she does not behave like a mother, then you are not at ease…if she begins to behave like a mother, then too you are not at ease.'

What is the solution? How to deal with children in such situations? Parents must learn to accept children in their uniqueness and appreciate their individuality without any judgement.

Joys of Bowing Down

In India, it is customary to touch the feet of religious gurus and the elderly. This training begins early when our parents force us to bow down whenever an elder person or a swami enters the house. Children usually hate doing this. This ritual is part of our social programming which has become a hypocritical exercise.

Respect for the elderly or swamis, bowing down to them or touching their feet, is a matter of sensitivity which gets corrupted when it is enforced. It should always be something natural—something done with feeling and understanding. When it is only a conditioning, a Hindu bows down to Hindu saints and a Muslim bows down to Muslim saints. Some people do bow down to all religious people; they too are conditioned to do that—out of fear or greed. Travelling around India in taxis or buses, I am always surprised to see drivers bow their heads to all kinds of temples on the roadside. It does not matter whether the place of worship belongs to Hindus or Muslims, whether it is some Baba's samadhi, a Sufi dargah or just a stone representing Hanumanji or a *Shivalinga*—these drivers bow down to all with equal respect.

Bowing down is something precious if it happens naturally. Bowing down to the rising or setting sun, the trees, the sky or the stars, connects us in some mysterious way to the universal energy that surrounds us all the time. This energy is divine and communing with this energy makes us feel divine. For a few moments, we become free from our ego. A man of sensitivity feels this all the time. In gratitude too, we become attuned to this cosmic energy.

In one of his *Darshan Diaries*, *The Tongue-Tip Taste of Tao*, Osho tells a seeker: 'I teach love for the world. Love this earth—it is really beautiful…it is utter splendour. Love from the smallest, the dewdrop, to the greatest star. Let this whole existence be your love object, let it be your beloved. Love has to be all-inclusive. And then only will you know the second thing, then only is the second possible—gratitude. Because when one is in love with existence one feels such blessing, such bliss, that it is natural to bow down in deep gratitude and when gratitude arises, prayer has arrived.' So remember these two things: Be loving and wait for gratitude to arrive.

The Temples of Love

You may have heard of an incident not so long ago when millions of people went to Allahabad for a holy dip in the Ganga. It was a gathering of the largest scale in India—really spectacular, though there was a tragic incident when many people died in a stampede at the railway station. It is a reality that at major religious events organised in Haridwar or Mecca, people get crushed and killed due to lack of discipline. Still people are drawn to these religious events.

The question is: Why do people go on pilgrimages where crowds are often unmanageable? To find peace, to sit and meditate and to feel the energy of those who have meditated there earlier. The power of collective prayer cannot be denied, even though the prayers may have their roots in greed to attain heaven and out of fear of hell after death. Today, most of the traditional temples have become centres of trade and politics. Regular prayers may be offered there but these prayers are just formal. There is no innocence in these prayers. In an atmosphere polluted with materialism and politics, meditation or true prayer is not possible.

If we are really interested in meditation and prayer, we need to look for a different kind of temple, one that is not man-made. And the good news is that such unpolluted temples of love still exist. You will find them in nature. Go and sit under a tree, breathe and meditate and you will be filled with love and prayer. The tree always gives life-energy. It will never ask you about your religion or caste. You can hug a tree and you will feel its heartbeat. At the same time, you will also feel your own heartbeat. But when you hug fellow human beings, you will not get the same feelings because nobody nowadays hugs anyone unconditionally. The tree is a temple of love, as it always gives.

Go to the mountains or the sea and sit in the open spaces. While you listen to the sound of mountains and streams, you will automatically start meditating. Meditation needs a certain kind of atmosphere, a space for the soul, where it can fly high in the sky. That is possible only in nature. Talking about the songs of the mystic saint Kabir, Osho says, 'To live with nature is to live with God in an indirect way because nature reflects God in a thousand and one ways. The trees and the call of the cuckoo and the winds in the pine trees and the rivers moving towards the ocean and the proud mountains standing in the sun and the starry night.... It is impossible not to be reminded of some invisible hands. The ocean heaves, breathes; the whole existence is a growing phenomenon. It is not dead, it cannot be dead. Everything is growing. Because of this growing experience man has remained constantly aware of some invisible, mysterious force behind it all. That force is called God. God is not a person but just a presence. Still when you go deep into the Himalayas, you again start feeling a kind of reverence, awe, wonder.'

Man is an emotional being. His mind is constantly swayed by all kinds of emotions, swinging from hate to love, jealousy to generosity and anger to compassion. Osho explains about an emotional personality: 'When it is anger, it is all anger and when it is love, it is all love. It almost becomes drunk with the emotion, blind and whatever action comes out of it is wrong. Whenever you are overwhelmed by any emotion you lose all reason, sensitivity. It becomes almost like a dark cloud in which you are lost.

Then whatever you do is going to be wrong.' This raises a question: Should we stop loving because it is an emotion? No. One can really love only when the love becomes more conscious and less emotional.

Osho says: 'Love is not to be a part of your emotions. Ordinarily that's what people think and experience but anything overwhelming is very unstable. It comes like a wind and passes by, leaving you behind, empty, shattered, in sadness and in sorrow. According to those who know man's whole being—his mind, his heart and his being—love has to be an expression of your being, not an emotion. Emotion is very fragile, very changing. One moment it seems that is all. Another moment you are simply empty.'

He suggests the first thing to do is to take love out of this crowd of overwhelming emotions. Love is not overwhelming. On the contrary, love is a tremendous insight, clarity, sensitivity and awareness. But that kind of love rarely exists because very few people ever reach to their being. We have to take love out from the emotional grip where it has been since our birth and we have to find a route to our being. Unless our love becomes part of our being, it is not much different from pain, suffering and sadness.

Osho has powerful methods of meditation to free us from overwhelming emotions, to unburden our heart. Through these meditations, we learn to transform the negative emotions into positive ones.

Love Will Cure This World!

The word 'belief' is capable of evoking evil as much as it is capable of doing good. But have we really bothered to sift our beliefs and choose what we believe in? If not, start right here. Believe in love, naturally....

George W Bush, the former president of the United States, wasn't a popular president. But he has been quite an entertainer because of his linguistic skills.

If you recall some of his statements—'I know what I believe. I will continue to articulate what I believe and what I believe—I believe what I believe is right'—they are hilariously funny. But to me, it is not just funny but profoundly absurd since his lines are based on the word belief. One can either know or believe. Because belief is generally borrowed—it is a piece of information acquired from other sources.

Priests are always asking us to believe in God. And people believe these beliefs without even experiencing God or godliness anywhere. Strangely, there are more definitions and beliefs than there are gods and believers choose and follow a definition of their choice. The trouble arises when they become staunch believers and start fighting about which definition is the ultimate. Such believers cannot tolerate other believers. And that is where the problem starts....

In one of his discourses, Osho says candidly: 'Belief is a dirty word! By belief you're prevented from knowing and you aren't helped. And it's because of beliefs; a man is divided as a Christian, a Hindu or a Muslim.

'It's belief that divides the world and creates wars. The moment you believe, you are no more one with humanity: You're a Christian, a Hindu or a Muslim. And you will be continuously fighting for your belief.'

Read this joke: A policeman was walking his beat when he saw two men fighting. A little boy was standing alongside and crying copiously, 'Daddy, Daddy!'

The officer pulled the two men apart and turning to the boy, asked, 'Which one is your father, lad?'

'I don't know,' the boy said, rubbing tears from his eyes, 'That's what they're fighting about.' Osho elaborates: 'Belief simply means you don't know, yet you believe. A blind man believing in light, what can belief do? He doesn't need a prophet or a messiah. What he needs is medicine or a surgeon for an eye operation so that he can see. And do you believe in light? Nobody asks such questions—you know light is there. The question of belief is asked only when the thing is nonexistential.'

In the name of religion or God, priests have been giving their followers belief systems which are inherently destructive. The real religious teaching can be only life affirmative, a true reverence for all life. The real religious teaching can only be of love. It cannot mislead the followers into killing other humans. But the priests provoke followers with ideologies and call it belief!

Osho says: 'Anybody who gives you a belief system is your enemy. You cannot see the truth and the desire to find truth disappears. But if all your belief systems are taken away from you, in the beginning, certainly it's bitter. I know the fear that will surface immediately. And only the search for truth and the experience of truth, not a belief is capable of healing your wounds.'

Cutting back to reality, the truth is in our heart, which is capable of healing not only our wounds but the cuts and bruises of this world. So, speak the language of the heart and learn to love, right away.... Will you?

Sufi Path of
Love—Fragrant and Fresh

Sufis tend to remain hidden in a mysterious world, revealing themselves only to the chosen seekers of truth, who are receptive and devoted. This has been their way for hundreds of years. They pray to God in the middle of the night, in its deep silence when the world sleeps as they do not want to flaunt their prayer.

In the Bhagavad Gita, Krishna says: 'The meditator meditates alone in the deep night when everybody in the world is sleeping.' Sufis do the same.

The story of Sufi Hakim Sanai, a Persian court poet, begins like a political thriller. He is moving with the Sultan of Persia and his military forces are on an expedition to conquer India. But as they pass a certain walled garden they come across a drunken singer, who is actually a great Sufi mystic, an enlightened man named Lai-Kur.

Osho says: 'Not much is known about Lai-Kur as people like him don't leave many footprints behind them. Except for this story, nothing has survived. But Lai-Kur continues to live in Sufi memory. Lai-Kur lives on the Everest of consciousness, way above the clouds.'

Only those who were fortunate and courageous enough to climb the mountain could comprehend his words. To the common masses, he was a madman. To knowers, he was just a vehicle of God and all that was coming through him was pure truth. Sufis remain in the world, they do not escape from it but deliberately they create a certain milieu around them so that people stop coming to them and they are left alone. Hakim Sanai was another such Sufi. His sayings are compiled in the *Hadiqa*, described by Osho as the essential fragrance of the path of love. Hakim Sanai has been able to catch the very soul of Sufism. Such books are not written, they are born; they come from the beyond, a gift. Their birth is as mysterious as that of a baby, a bird or a rose.

Osho says: 'Hakim Sanai, this name is as sweet to me as honey, as sweet as nectar. He is unique in the world of Sufism. No other Sufi has been able to reach to such heights of expression and such depths of penetration.' The poem of Hakim Sanai reveals the profundity of his mystic thought:

> We tried reasoning
> Our way to him
> It didn't work;
> But the moment we gave up,
> No obstacle remained.
> He introduced himself to us
> Out of kindness: How else
> Could we have known him?
> Reason took us as far as the door;
> But it was his presence that let us in.
> But how will you ever know him,
> As long as you are unable
> To know yourself
> Once one is one,
> No more, no less
> Error begins with duality.

Osho explains: 'Reason is not the only door in your being; there are deeper doors in your being. Can't you feel the beat of the heart? When you look at a lotus flower and you feel the beauty, is it reason? Can reason prove that the flower is beautiful? Reason has not even been able to define what beauty is. For the rational mind, there is no beauty. But you know that beauty exists and when you see it, you are overwhelmed by it. The rational mind says there is no beauty; this is just an illusion, a projection, a dream. Beauty exists. But reason has no way to approach it; it is felt from the heart. Love exists; that too is not through reason, that too is felt from the heart. When you fall in love, can you justify it rationally? Can you say what love is? Nobody has yet been able to. God is all these experiences together: The experience of beauty, the experience of good, the experience of love, the experience of truth. All these experiences happen through the heart. The totality of these experiences is called God.'

Discover True Love

While everybody in the world is seeking love to nourish one's being and soul, people end up having all kinds of troubles and misfortunes because of love. Everybody desires nectar but gets poison in the name of love. Everyone wonders how that happens. What is the answer? What is the solution? Is it possible to find love in the true sense?

Many sages, philosophers, psychologists, priests and other people have tried their best to enlighten us on this issue and most of us have been following their advice. But the advice does not work. It does not work because the source of the advice is outside us—it is not arising from our own heart. Our heart, if it functions properly, if it is open and sensitive, can show us the way to love. But the trouble is that the social atmosphere in which we are brought up is not conducive to this. It is filled with doubt and fear. It would be a real miracle to maintain the original purity of our heart in such an atmosphere.

A child comes out of the womb and enters the world with all the trust. There is the mother to feed him and look after his needs. The mother showers her unconditional love on the child. The child grows up beautifully, feeling trust and love. But when he enters the world, goes beyond the confines of the immediate family, the child does not find the same atmosphere. It is quite the opposite—ambition, competition, doubt, fear, conflict and violence confront him. It begins with education where a child is taught to compete and be at the top of the class. Unthinkingly, his own family also starts supporting this ambition.

This certainly is not the way of the heart—it kills the heart gradually. When the child grows up, he falls in love. This is not the same love that he had received as an infant. Now the love has become contaminated with ambition and competition, doubt and fear. This is going to reflect in his new love-relationships. After a few years, the relationship will stagnate. The heart will be dominated by the mind, contaminated by social corruption. Love will evaporate in such storms and life will become miserable. In such a situation, life can only go downhill.

If a man is able to protect his consciousness from this polluting social atmosphere, he will seek meditation and spirituality to raise his consciousness. Only such a consciousness will show him the way to pure love. Meditation will create a bridge between him and the universe and he will get the same motherly love on a higher level. When there is faith, the whole existence functions as a mother.

Osho says: 'You are not accidental. Existence needs you. Without you, something will be missing in existence and nobody can replace it. That's what gives you dignity, that the whole existence will miss you. The stars and sun and moon and birds and earth—everything in the universe will feel a small place is vacant which cannot be filled by anybody except you. This gives you a tremendous joy, a fulfilment that you are related to existence and existence cares for you. Once you are clean and clear, you will receive tremendous love from all directions.'

Nature is a Celebration

An enlightened mystic J Krishnamurti did not wear the traditional clothes of a sadhu or a sannyasi. He did not have a beard of a sage or shaved head of a Buddhist monk.

He had no hypocrisy of any kind. He did not create any image about himself and led a simple life with all the grace of an awakened one—a Buddha. His crystal-clear message of awareness is central to his teachings. He talks about his own being in some poetic words which reads like a sutra from some Upanishad: 'I have no name. I am as the fresh breeze of the mountains. I have no shelter; I am as the wandering waters. I have no sanctuary like the dark Gods, nor am I in the shadow of deep temples. I have no sacred books, nor am I well-seasoned in tradition. I am neither in the graven image, nor in the rich chant of a melodious voice. I am not bound by theories, nor corrupted by beliefs. I am not held by the bondage of religions, nor in the pious agony of their priests. I am not entrapped by philosophies, nor held in the power of their sects. I am neither low nor high. I am the worshipper and the worshipped. I am free. My song is the song of the river, calling for the open seas. Wandering, I am life. I have no name; I am as the fresh breeze of the mountains.'

This is the ultimate expression of an enlightened person, who has no identification with any worldly image. His consciousness is not contaminated or conditioned by the various belief systems imposed on him. He is pure as Gangotri, the original source of the river Ganga descending from the Himalayas. This river has the absolute freedom of flowing to reach the ocean. It carries no road maps to follow certain instructions to reach its destination. It is destined to reach its goal with its natural flow, without any push or support system. It does not pray to any God as it does not feel any separation from God. It is in bliss of being itself—the bliss of freedom.

We, human beings, with all kinds of support systems of belief and social conditioning, live a life of imprisonment created by our own thoughts and worries. Society and religion make us afraid of hell and greedy for heaven. Living this way, we feel vulnerable and insecure and we create a certain shell around ourselves. This shell is our personality, which is the result of fear and greed. Gradually, we so fully identify with this imaginary image that it becomes our reality and we forget our real being. Then we spend our lives fighting to protect this pseudo-being. All our sufferings are born out of our living this unnatural way. We lose connection or communion with our inner nature leading to disconnect with nature outside us—the earth, the sky, the sun, the moon and the stars.

Osho says, 'If you can trust nature, by and by you become quiet, silent, happy, joyful, celebrating because nature is celebrating. Nature is a celebration. Look all around. Can you see any flower which looks like your saints? Can you see any rainbow which looks like your saints? Or any cloud, bird singing and the light reflecting in the river and the stars? The world is celebrating. The world is not sad. The world is a song, an utterly beautiful song and the dance continues. Become part of this dance and trust your nature. If you trust your nature, you will come closer to the cosmic nature. That is the only way. You are part of the cosmic. When you trust yourself, you have trusted the cosmic in you. From that small thread, you can reach the very goal. Trusting yourself, you have trusted God who has made you. Not trusting yourself, you have distrusted God who has made you.'

Sing a Song, Sing Out Loud!

For those who are spiritual, religion becomes a serious affair as they think they are doing something holy by following certain rituals. They start feeling holier than others, superior to others. This creates an ego, an image, a false identity and often people go astray from true religiousness and their authentic being.

Their mind becomes more dominant than the heart. The mind is full of thoughts while the heart is full of love, compassion and sensitivity. Sometimes the heart can act so irrationally that the mind may not understand it.

There is a story of St Francis of Assisi, who sang while lying on his deathbed. He sang so loudly that the entire neighbourhood could hear him.

Brother Elias, a pompous but prominent member of the Franciscan Order, came close to St Francis and said, 'Father, there are people standing in the street outside your window. I am afraid nothing we might do could prevent them from hearing you singing. The lack of restraint at so grave an hour might embarrass the Order, Father. It might lower the esteem in which you yourself are so justly held. Perhaps you have lost sight of your obligation to those who have come to regard you as a saint. Would it not be more edifying for them if you would, err, die with more Christian dignity?'

'Please excuse me, Brother,' St Francis said, 'But I feel so much joy in my heart that I really can't help it. I must sing!' And he died singing.

In his discourse on the *Diamond Sutra*, Osho explains this: 'Brother Elias wanted to prove to people that St Francis is a saint. He was afraid about what would people think of St Francis—they may think he was mad.

'A saint has to be serious by the very definition...Brother Elias was worried that St Francis would leave a bad name. People might either think that he was not a saint or he was mad. But in reality, Brother Elias was not worried about St Francis; he was worried about himself and the Order.

'Brother Elias wanted to prove that his master was the greatest master. And he knew only one way to prove it—that he should become serious, he should take life seriously, he should not laugh and should not sing and dance.

'These things are too human, they are too ordinary. Ordinary mortals can be forgiven but not a man of the stature of St Francis.

'But St Francis had a different vision—he was "ordinary". At the time of dying, the self, the ego did not exist. St Francis did not exist as an individual.

'There was absolute silence and peace within him. Out of that silence, the song was born. What could St Francis have done?'

Osho concludes: 'There can be no other better death than that of St Francis. If you can die singing that proves that you lived singing; your life was a joy and death became its crescendo, the culmination. St Francis is a Buddha. The characteristic of a Buddha is that he is ordinary, that he has no ideas about himself of how he should be, that he simply is spontaneous, that whatsoever happens, happens. He lives at the spur of the moment.'

Talking in Tongues

An ambitious, fast-paced life full of competition gives sleepless nights to many around the world. Our unnatural lifestyle and overactive mind does not let us have sound sleep at night. As a result, we often see people becoming increasingly dependent on all kinds of intoxicants, drugs and sleeping pills. This is very dangerous.

A recently published study suggests that sleeping pills taken by tens of thousands of Britons can increase the risk of heart attack by up to 50 per cent. Scientists have found that zolpidem, which is sold under the brand name Stilnoct in the UK, is linked with a dramatic rise in the number of life-threatening cardiac ailments. The study—presented at the world's biggest cardiology conference—is the first to connect the drug with cardiovascular problems. So is there any meditative solution for sleeplessness? Yes, there is and it does not cost anything. Every night, before going to bed, one simply needs to declutter one's mind. How does one declutter the mind?

Osho explains: 'Every night, before you go to sleep, put the lights out and sit on your bed for fifteen minutes. Close your eyes and then start humming any monotonous sound, for example, "la, la, la" and then wait for the mind to supply new sounds. The only thing to remember is that those sounds or words should not be of any language that you understand. Speak any language that you do not know. For a few seconds, you may find it difficult but it can be done. Once your mind starts coming up with random sounds and nonsense words, your conscious mind will be off. Your unconscious mind is speaking.

'When the unconscious speaks, it knows no language. It is a very old method. It comes from the Old Testament. In those days it was called "glossolalia", and a few churches in America still use it. They call it "talking in tongues". And it is a wonderful method.

'These fifteen minutes will relax the conscious mind deeply. Then you can just lie down and go to sleep. Your sleep will become deeper. Within weeks, you will feel a depth in your sleep and in the morning, you will feel fresh.

'This may sound bizarre but this technique really works. The modern man lives life at a maddening speed that cannot be called sane. For a mad lifestyle, some methods of conscious madness are really useful.

'During the entire day, we spend so much time watching television and feeding our mind with all kinds of garbage that is dished out. The scenes of politicians fighting with each other endlessly, the saddening news of rape and violence overburden our mind. If we carry this weight into our sleep, we cannot expect to have a restful mind and good sleep. We need to empty our mind of all the rubbish before entering our inner being.'

Negativity is the Root of Illness

Ralph Waldo Emerson wrote: 'To be yourself in a world that is constantly trying to make you something else is the greatest accomplishment.'

Every child who enters this world faces this dilemma. Parents start moulding the child with all good intentions in accordance with their religious beliefs and culture. When the child grows up, he desires to understand life the way he sees it. But it is difficult for him to view life with a purity of consciousness. He is not free to experiment. Parents, elders and teachers do not allow him the freedom to explore. Many things are imposed on the child's psyche and the child eventually starts losing his individuality and starts developing into an unoriginal and unauthentic personality.

Instead of growing up to be a unique human being, he develops a persona as desired and expected by his elders. Then begins the endless conflict between his unique individuality and his moulded personality. This is the root cause of disease.

The author of *Dying To Be Me*, Anita Moorjani, has lived a life of torture, fear and guilt. This social suffocation took the form of cancer in her body and being. She was often asked why she got cancer and she would sum up her answer in one word: Fear.

She writes: 'What was I afraid of? Just about everything including failing, being disliked, letting people down and not being good enough. I also feared illness, cancer in particular, as well as the treatment for cancer. I was afraid of living and I was afraid of dying.

'Fear is very subtle and it can creep up gradually without our even noticing it. Looking back, I see that most of us are taught from a very young age to be afraid, although I don't believe we're born this way.'

True, nobody is born this way. Every child comes into the world as tabula rasa—a blank slate. So whatever his parents, teachers, priests write on him, the child starts seeing it as destiny, as fate.

The child comes into this world with all doors, directions and dimensions throbbing to be explored. But before the child can choose or learn to comprehend the feel of his being, he is corrupted and the psyche is polluted.

There are preachers who teach the child to become God-fearing. Such preachers have been exploiting their followers with fear and greed. It is very rare to find somebody teaching people to be God-loving or teaching love for life—the real nourishment for the soul.

Osho tried to liberate people from this negative attitude—the root cause of most illnesses and, maybe, even cancer. Accepting oneself and loving oneself, without any fear or guilt, opens the doors to good health and godliness. Being in harmony with oneself is the way to be in harmony with the whole existence.

Osho says: 'My whole teaching is—just be yourself, never interfere with anybody else's freedom. Freedom is my ultimate value.... Harmony is happiness and harmony is heaven. And harmony happens only when you are in tune with the whole. To be with the whole is to be holy.... The moment you experience your own being, you have experienced the being of this whole universe because your heartbeat is part of the heartbeat of the universe.'

The Boat is Empty

I have seen many people getting possessed by strong emotions and it takes a while to be free from their poisonous effect. It is not just about our major conflicts with people; even insignificant things may trigger something in our unconscious mind that may lead to big emotional explosions.

In such moments, we become helpless and we start getting angry at others who may be totally innocent. We become angry even at inanimate things. Many people, when they are in some kind of rage, find themselves pushing or banging a door, venting their anger on the door.

How to deal with such clumsy situations?

There is an insight about this in a Zen story: A great Zen master, Lin Chi, used to say, 'While I was young I was very fascinated by boating. I had one small boat and I would go on the lake alone. For hours together I would remain there. One night, I was meditating in my boat. One empty boat came floating downstream and struck my boat. My eyes were closed, so I thought someone is here with his boat and has struck my boat. Anger arose. I opened my eyes and I was just about to utter something to that man in anger, when I realised that the boat was empty. To whom should I express my anger? The boat was empty and was just floating downstream.

So there was nothing to do. There was no possibility to project anger on an empty boat.'

So Lin Chi said, 'The anger was there but finding no way out, I closed my eyes and just floated backward with the anger. And that empty boat became my realisation. I came to a point within myself. That empty boat was my master. And now if someone comes and insults me, I laugh and I say, "This boat is also empty." I close my eyes and I go within.'

Osho provides a powerful method to deal with strong emotions: 'Just a simple phenomenon has to be learnt—I call it meditation. It has been called by different names. Lord Buddha used to call it *sammasati*, right mindfulness. The Armenian spiritual teacher, George Gurdjieff, called it self-remembering. The whole thing is how to become a witness.

'When you are angry, there is no need to fight with it—it is a great opportunity to watch. No need to indulge in it, no need to act according to it and no need either to go to the opposite extreme and start fighting with it. Avoid both. Just remain cool, detached, a simple observer as if it has nothing to do with you. Your concern should be scientific; you are observing, so you have to look minutely at what anger is in all its details, in its whole mystery. Your interest has to be scientific—you have to go deeper into the whole method of it. If you follow it, you will not be able to go into it. You will become angry. In that hot state, how can you watch? If you fight with it again, it will be the same: You will be running away, repressing, avoiding. How can you watch something of which you are afraid?

'No need to be afraid, no need to follow—just sit silently and watch and a miracle starts happening slowly: The more you watch, the more you see that it is dispersing on its own. Just as dewdrops evaporate in the morning sun, it starts evaporating faster as your awareness becomes more intense.'

Live Life the Feminine Way

There are two fundamental ways of living our life—one is the masculine way and the other is the feminine way. Though both the ways are opposite to each other, yet they are complementary.

The masculine way is aggressive while the feminine way is receptive. The masculine way may seem very strong and powerful but it is not the existential reality, which is quite mysterious. The enlightened mystics such as Krishna, Buddha, Lao Tzu and many others who radiate so much feminine grace, praise the feminine power.

Lao Tzu says:

> *The valley spirit, undying*
> *Is called the Mystic Female*
> *The gate of the Mystic Female*
> *Is called the root of Heaven and Earth*
> *It flows continuously, barely perceptible*
> *Utilise it; it is never exhausted.*

The way of the Tao is the way of the feminine—delicate yet very powerful, soft yet strong, passive yet irresistible, illogical yet magical. This is quite difficult for man to understand. He finds that there's something so mysterious about woman that he cannot fathom it. Man is born out of a woman; he lives all his life with her, even then what is that something within a woman that is forever strange and unknown to man?

This very element in the woman is what Lao Tzu calls the Valley Spirit. It is not something logical or rational—it is suprarational. This is the beauty of life. Life becomes utterly boring if we can understand everything about it. Life is not mathematical. But a man's mind easily understands things that are mathematical. And things which are not understandable by the mind are considered complicated.

He cannot understand the ways of the woman. That's why most of the man–woman relationships become complicated and end in fights.

The feminine way of looking at life or living life is less calculative and more mysterious, less logical and more lovable. That is why the wise people tell us: Do not try to understand women—just love them. The same insight is equally true about life: Try not to understand it—just live it and love it. Live it intensely and love it deeply.

Osho explains it beautifully: 'A woman is to be loved, not understood.' That is the first understanding. Life is so mysterious that our hands cannot reach up to its heights; our eyes cannot look into its deepest mystery. Understanding any expression of existence is the function of science, not of a mystic.

With Albert Einstein, the whole history of science has taken a very different route because the more he went into the deepest core of matter, the more he became puzzled. Existence does not follow logic. Logic is man-made. A point comes when you have to abandon logic and rationality and just listen to nature.

I call it the ultimate understanding but not in the ordinary sense of understanding. You know it, you feel it but there is no way to say it.

Live Life in its Totality

Talking about the four noble truths, the Buddha is reported to have said, *Jeevan dukkha hai* (life is suffering or misery). *Dukkha* means a lot of things. For example, anything temporary can be *dukkha* including happiness; anything that is impermanent, illusory can be *dukkha*.

People argue about this statement and say that it a very depressing statement by an enlightened master. It is. But it is also a fact of life. For some people, life may not be so full of misery but for the majority of people it is. One does not have to be too sensitive to see or feel it, it is all around us. It is there even in the rich Western society. In spite of all the wealth and scientific progress, we have not been able to live happily and in harmony with our relationships and the rest of the world. The outer richness has not solved the inner misery and darkness. Everybody is in some kind of despair and pain. It is no use going into all kinds of details of suffering and misery of life, it is much better to find a way to end it as soon as possible by going beyond it.

Osho gives us a simple method of transforming pain into compassion. It is a breathing technique. He says, 'When you breathe in, imagine that you are breathing in all the darkness and negativity in your life. Welcome it into your heart. Stop trying to resist, avoid or destroy it. That has been taking up all of your energy. As you are breathing in this heaviness, let it be absorbed into your heart before you exhale. And then the moment you breathe out, breathe out golden light. Breathe out your greatest lightness, your highest joy, love and blessing from your heart into the source of the negativity. You will soon transform all the darkness in your life with your breath. Breathe out all the love that you have, all the blissfulness that you have, all the benediction that you have. When breathing out, pour your love into existence. This is the method of compassion: Drink in all the suffering and pour out all the blessings. And you will be surprised what happens when you really do it. The moment you stop resisting all the darkness and heaviness in your inner world, there is no longer suffering. The heart has the power to transform any energy to light. The heart is the essential alchemist. It can drink in any misery, pain or sadness and transform it into lightness. Trust the power of your heart. Once you have learned that your heart can do this magic, this miracle, keep practising it again and again. Experiment with this exercise and let yourself explore every dark area of your life. If you feel overwhelmed, don't give up. It is often the coldest and darkest just before dawn. Just let yourself fully feel that which you cannot feel, what you've been resisting. Only then will you have mastered yourself. Continue doing this beautiful method of transforming pain into compassion for thirty days. You'll get better at it and be able to welcome in all the heaviness of the world and pour out such great love and light that our entire planet will be transformed. You have the power within you to do miracles, use it! You'll see how amazingly bright, brilliant and alive you will feel!'

Being alive means that you are full of energy and then your life is no more a suffering but a blessing. This blessedness does not happen in isolation—it is a sharing of bliss. It is a celestial party. Osho illustrates this with a beautiful parable: 'In paradise one afternoon, in its most famous café, Lao Tzu, Confucius and the Buddha are sitting and chatting. The waiter comes with a tray that holds three glasses of juice called "life" and offers it to them. The Buddha immediately closes his eyes and refuses, he says, "Life is misery". Lao Tzu takes all the three glasses and he says, "Unless one drinks totally, how can one say anything?" Lao Tzu drinks all the three glasses and starts dancing! The Buddha and Confucius ask him, "Are you not going to say anything?" And Lao Tzu says, "This is what I am saying—my dance and my song are speaking for me." Unless you taste totally, you cannot say. And when you taste totally, you still cannot say because what you know is such that no words are adequate. The Buddha is at one extreme, Confucius is in the middle. Lao Tzu has drunk all the three glasses—the one that was brought for the Buddha, the one that was brought for Confucius and the one that was brought for him. He has drunk them all; he has lived life in its three-dimensionality.'

Osho declares, 'My own approach is that of Lao Tzu. Live life in all possible ways; don't choose one thing against the other and don't try to be in the middle. Don't try to balance yourself—balance is not something that can be cultivated. Balance is something that comes out of experiencing all the dimensions of life. Balance is something that happens; it is not something that can be brought about through your efforts. If you bring it through your efforts it will be false, forced. And you will remain tense; you will not be relaxed because how can a person who is trying to remain balanced in the middle be relaxed? You will always be afraid that if you relax, you may start moving to the left or to the right. You are bound to remain uptight and to be uptight is to miss the whole opportunity, the whole gift of life. Don't be uptight. Don't live life according to principles. Live life in its totality, drink life in its totality! Yes, sometimes it tastes bitter—so what? That taste of bitterness will make you capable of tasting its sweetness. You will be able to appreciate the sweetness only if you have tasted its bitterness. One who knows not how to cry will not know how to laugh either. One who cannot enjoy a deep laughter, a belly laugh, that person's tears will be crocodile tears. They cannot be true, they cannot be authentic.'

A Life of Beauty

Beauty is truth's smile
when she beholds her own face in a perfect mirror.

Beauty is in the ideal of perfect harmony
which is in the universal being,
truth the perfect comprehension of the universal mind.

—Rabindranath Tagore

On 7 May we celebrate the birthday of our greatest poet Rabindranath Tagore, who was also a mystic, a rishi and above all, a worshipper of beauty.

The enlightened mystics of India have defined the ultimate experience as *Satyam, Shivam* and *Sundaram*—Truth, goodness and beauty. The beauty comes after truth and goodness. But for this mystic poet, beauty came first. He loved beauty so much that he would not have chosen truth and goodness if they were without beauty. This is what made him unique and outstanding. The moralists may not have agreed with his attitude but that did not create any guilt in Rabindranath. He continued to follow his heart that loved beauty more than anything else. Rabindranath was a spiritualist in his own way. He did not pray in temples or followed any traditional rituals though he was born a Hindu. He cannot be confined to a certain section of humanity. He belongs to *Vasudhaiva Kutumbakam*—the whole earth is one family. The same way he cannot be confined to India though he was born in this country. He was a world-traveller who loved to be a wanderer. He was also educated in the West, yet, he had deep roots in India. He was truly a world citizen born in India.

His greatest contribution is his poems in *Gitanjali—Song Offerings*. He used to say that he had nothing else to offer. 'I am just as poor as a bird or as rich as a bird. I can sing a song every morning fresh and new, in gratefulness. I want to offer God exactly what is my heartbeat. I don't want to be a believer; I want to be a knower. I don't want to be knowledgeable; I want to be innocent enough so that existence reveals its mysteries to me. I don't want to be worshipped as a saint.'

Paying tribute to him, Osho says: 'And the fact is that in this whole century, there was nobody else more saintly than Rabindranath Tagore but he refused to be recognised as a saint. He said, "I have only one desire—to be remembered as a singer of songs, as a dancer, as a poet who has offered all his potential, all his flowers of being, to the unknown divineness of existence. I don't want to be worshipped; I consider it a humiliation...ugly, inhuman and removed from the world completely. Every man contains God; every cloud, every tree, every ocean is full of godliness, so who is to worship whom?"'

This is the beauty of the mystic poet which transcends all traditional concepts of religion and spirituality. Osho adores him and makes the spirit of Rabindranath alive in the following words:

'Look at the trees, look at the birds, look at the clouds, look at the stars and if you have eyes, you will be able to see that the whole existence is joyful. Everything is simply happy. Trees are happy for no reason; they are not going to become prime ministers or presidents and they are not going to become rich and they will never have any bank balance. Look at the flowers—for no reason. It is simply unbelievable how happy flowers are.'

An Effort to Live

Terrorism is wrong! We all know that but how are we planning to curb it? If fighting is our only antidote, it is not right either. Fight yourself first. Start this change...Now!

India had witnessed some ghastly acts of terror—the decadence of the human spirit or shall I say insanity to end lives for the sake of the most abused word in the world, religion.

Amidst all this bloodbath, lies an eternal question: Can we put an end to terrorism? Or will we continue to live helplessly and hopelessly? Is there no solution at hand or is there...can't we transform ourselves and change our environment in the process?

I'm not saying all this to tell the world that I know of any real solution. Because since time immemorial, terrorism has been an all-pervasive phenomenon. And it seems it may never end, even with the promises and rhetoric by politicians. Because the truth is that even they aren't secure, are they?

Yet, there is something we can do to change the situation by transforming our own lives for the better. For example, when Angulimala met Gautama Buddha, the enlightened one, just meeting him transformed his life. The Buddha became a catalyst and it was his presence that awakened Angulimala to his misdeeds. Similarly, we can awaken the Buddha within us—we have seeds of Buddhahood just as we have seeds of terrorism inside us. What seeds we nurture within our lives always depends on us. Everybody, each one of us, has both kinds of seeds—terrorism and consciousness.

Osho tells an anecdote from Buddha's life. 'Once a farmer asked the Buddha, "Why don't you do something? I cultivate land while you simply sit under the tree with eyes closed, doing nothing. I have been watching you, people come to you, you talk to them and sometimes they silently sit by your side. Why don't you do something?"

The poor farmer was naturally curious since he had been watching Buddha under a tree, doing no work at all.

The Buddha replied, "Can't you see I'm also a farmer? My farm is of a different quality and on a different plane. I grow the crop of bliss. I sow the seeds of bliss. The people who come around and sit silently or to whom sometimes I talk—they are my work, I am sowing seeds in people's consciousness. In the right season they will bloom. I've bloomed and cultivated my inner soil. Now my soul is full of flowers!"'

Osho helps us realise this pure presence of our own beings. He says: 'To me, that is liberation. To me, that is the ultimate flowering of your being. Your eyes will show it, your hands will indicate it, your dance may become a part of the overflow. You will be a transformed human being.'

And at this juncture of time, we need millions of transformed beings who can fill the world with joy and roses of consciousness. With the light of awareness, with the music of soul. Because only that can prevent the politicians from destroying this world. Perhaps you may not have noted but destruction also gives a certain power. Just as creation gives tremendous well-being and dignity.... Those who cannot create have only engaged in destruction sometimes in the name of politics or religion or education or anything else.

So, the only way to build a beautiful and peaceful world is to create a force of creative people. Those who can create more than they can destroy. Be the change you want to see!

Excellence in Life

Difficulties are like divine surgery, do not resist them. Nature expects us to use our heart and head to discover new and wiser skills to fly in life.

Observe the commitment of an eagle in bringing out excellence while choosing a partner first and parenting later. An eagle tests before it trusts. Before mating, a female eagle tests its partner. It picks up a twig, flies high and as the male follows, it flies around to escape and finally drops the twig. Before the twig falls on the ground, the male catches the twig and gives it to the female. It repeats this act. If a male succeeds in catching the twig consistently, then it allows mating to take place.

Similarly, like an eagle, can we test before we trust? Eagles lay eggs on a cliff by making a nest of grass entwined with thorns. When the eggs hatch, the weight of the eaglets makes the female eagle uncomfortable as the thorns start pricking. Then the female pushes the eaglets out of the nest. As the eaglets are about to fall, the male picks them up. Meanwhile, the female removes the upper layer of grass, so that the eaglets rest directly on the thorns. The eaglets are yet to test their wings to fly. Now the male pushes the eaglets out of the nest. This process continues till such time that the eaglets are able to foresee the danger in falling and start using their wings. Bring similar commitment to all walks of life.

Excellence happens when there is love to grow and contribute. Intention leads to creativity. Intention is like sowing a seed in existence—you allow it to germinate and let the forces of nature nurture life.

Commitment also involves dropping illusions. We do not see the world as it is. We see the world projected through our verbose minds. Minds are filled with thoughts, which are nothing but mere words. Words represent experiences. Words are also influenced by memory. Memory is of the past. From the past, we see the present. Hence, we create illusions created by words but we must filter them wisely.

The mind creates dreams. The self-awareness in you sees reality. Awareness without the arrogant 'I' is the 'higher self'. The mind with its illusions is the 'lower self'. Have the commitment to operate from the 'higher self'.

Through commitment, balance all walks of your life. Creativity is to balance your life and move on to excellence.

Mystics and Beards

On my recent trip to the United States, a man working in a restaurant greeted me with '*Assalamualaikum*' and I responded with '*Waalaikumassalaam*'. In a shop in New York, the shopkeeper, perhaps an Indian or Pakistani, told me that he would give me a big discount as I was a Muslim. In both the places, I wondered why they thought of me as a Muslim.

Perhaps my small beard and kurta–pajama gave the impression that I was a Muslim. In India, I have never been considered a Muslim—only in the United States. This was a bit strange for me but I loved it.

It is natural that most people look at others with their own limited understanding and that is perhaps why the beard, which has nothing to do with any particular religion, has come to be identified with one. You can have a beard without belonging to any religion.

Down the ages, only religious people, artists, poets and philosophers had beards. Other regular people shaved it off routinely. Sages and Hindu and Sikh gurus were known for their long beards. It was important to have a beard to be seen as a guru or a wise man. In recent times, J Krishnamurti, Meher Baba and Ramana Maharishi did not have beards, yet they were the enlightened masters.

J Krishnamurti wore western clothes and a necktie in the West and kurta–pajama in India, and he looked very handsome in both. Osho had a long beard and wore long, flowing robes. Rabindranath Tagore, who was addressed as Gurudev, had the same kind of flowing beard.

It is believed that wise men always have long, grey beards so people who want to seem wise, usually grow one. At least, the wise men of Islam, Judaism and Greek Orthodox Christianity did so. The Pope is clean-shaven, because Roman Catholic clergy shave as a sign of celibacy. Confucius had a beard and he was wise too. Santa Claus has a beautiful beard and children love him.

I have also heard that the Bible has a commandment against shaving—actually against touching the razor to the face. So Jews, who religiously follow the Bible, do not touch the razor to the face. In modern times, it is possible to shave without a razor touching the face and many do so. Sikhs do not cut their hair, so the beard sort of happens by default.

During one of Osho's discourses, a disciple asked an interesting question: 'Last night, I noticed your beard. It is really a magnificent thing; it reminds me of a lion's mane. Does a beard like yours come with enlightenment? Or do you have to be born with it?'

Osho replied: 'You are a little bit crazy but not more than me. I insist: If you want this kind of beard, you will have to be born with it. It does not come with enlightenment. Enlightenment has no concern with your beard. Even a woman can become enlightened. That does not mean she will have a beard. This kind of beautiful beard comes only with your birth.'

The Divine Within

All over the world, people say hello when they greet each other but in India we greet each other with namaste or namaskar. This means: I bow down to the divine within you. In the modern times, this greeting has become as formal as the fake smile one gets from air hostesses. With namaste, namaskar or hello, people do not feel the warmth towards each other; greeting has become a formality or a ritual. Otherwise, this simple gesture can help us live a happy and harmonious life. We greet each other but live in all sorts of conflicts.

There is a very meaningful Zen story that teaches a divine way of solving our conflicts at the workplace or even at home.

The abbot of a once famous Buddhist monastery, that gradually started declining, was deeply troubled. Monks were lax in their practice, novices were leaving and lay supporters were abandoning the monastery. He travelled far to a sage and recounted his tale of woe—of how much he desired to transform his monastery into a flourishing haven it had been in days of yore. The sage looked at him and said, 'The reason your monastery has languished is that the Buddha is living among you in disguise and you have not honoured Him.'

The abbot hurried back, his mind in turmoil. The Selfless One was at his monastery! Who could He be? Brother Hua? No, he was full of sloth. Brother Po? No, he was too dull. He summoned all the monks and revealed the sage's words. They, too, were taken aback and looked at each other with suspicion and awe. Which one of them was the Chosen One? The disguise was perfect. Not knowing who He was, they took to treating everyone with the respect due to Gautama Buddha. Their faces started shining with an inner radiance that attracted novices and then other supporters. In no time, the monastery far surpassed its previous glory.

The enlightened mystics have always taught us to see the divine in every human being or every living being. But our mind is always suspicious. Everybody in this world seems to be our competitor of some sort. So, instead of working in harmony with each other and sharing our joy with all, we start living in a private world of our own.

This way we create our mental prisons and become confined to a limited self while we are designed by existence to transcend our limits.

The Zen teaches us to be free from such psychological confinements. It does not teach ordinary freedom, it teaches us the ultimate freedom: Freedom from oneself. We are in the bondage of our limited self, the prison of our ego which does not tolerate inclusion of others. It perceives others as others. Remember the famous quote of Jean Paul Sartre: 'The other is hell.'

Osho says, 'To see other as the other is hell.' He reminds us: 'Hell and heaven are within you. The doors are very close: With the right hand you can open one, with the left hand you can open another. With just a change of your mind, your being is transformed—from heaven to hell and from hell to heaven. This goes on continuously. What is the secret? The secret is whenever you are unconscious, whenever you act unconsciously, without awareness, you are in hell; whenever you are conscious, whenever you act with full awareness, you are in heaven. If this awareness becomes so integrated, so consolidated, that you never lose it, there is no hell for you; if unconsciousness becomes so consolidated, so integrated, that you never lose it, there is no heaven.'

Laugh Your Way to God

Down the centuries, religion has been a very serious affair for most believers. It was too ritualistic and grim. Being pious or holy became synonymous with seriousness. Hence, the so-called religion deprived people of their natural innocent laughter. By performing so many rituals, people became egoistical, while the priests and the religious followers started feeling holier than others. This conduct made them hypocrites and forbidding.

Gradually, the whole affair of religion became heavy and morose and most of the people have been living with that burden on their heart. They forgot to laugh and celebrate. Osho observed all these and said: 'All over the world, sadness has become so prominent. And temples and churches don't look festive, they don't give a sense of celebration. Religion cannot be anything other than a celebration of life.... A man too much burdened by theories becomes serious. A man who is unburdened, has no burden of theories over his being, starts laughing.'

Osho introduced laughter as a process of unburdening the conditioned mind. During one of his discourses on the *Akshya Upanishad*, he explained the significance of laughter in human life: 'There are three types of laughter. The first is when you laugh at someone else. This is the meanest, the lowest, the most ordinary and vulgar. This is the violent, aggressive and insulting type. Deep down in this laughter, there is always a feeling of revenge.

'The second type of laughter is when you laugh at yourself. This is worth achieving. This is cultured. And a man who can laugh at himself is valuable. He has risen above vulgarity. He has risen above lowly instincts—hatred, aggression, violence.

'And the third is the last and the highest. This is not about anybody, neither about oneself nor the other. It is just cosmic. You laugh at the whole situation as it is. The whole situation of existence is such that if you can see the whole—such a great infinite vastness moving toward no fixed purpose, no goal—laughter will arise. So much is going on without leading anywhere; nobody is there in the past to create it; nobody is there in the future to finish it. Such is the whole cosmos. If you can see this whole cosmos, then laughter is inevitable.'

Laughter relaxes. And relaxation is spiritual. Laughter brings you to the earth, brings you down from your stupid ideas of being holier than thou. Laughter brings you to reality, as it is. The world is a playground of God, a cosmic joke. And unless you understand it as a cosmic joke, you will never be able to understand the ultimate mystery.

Rage Rooms and Meditation

As the modern civilisation becomes more and more uncivilised, some intelligent people around the world are becoming concerned and looking for solutions to bring in some sanity. The whole world seems to be going mad—people are in a real rage and the volcanoes of anger and violence are erupting almost daily.

Recently, two Serbian teenagers set up a 'Rage Room' where people can vent their anger and frustration by destroying things. Customers are handed a baseball and a hard bat before they unleash their anger on lamps, beds, tables and other pieces of furniture. The 'Rage Room' has drawn a flurry of attention since it opened in the northern Serbian city of Novi Sad, where two decades of war, political crisis and economic hardship have driven many people over the edge.

Travelling around the world, I noticed that at all the major airports, there are prayer rooms for believers of different religions. The airports of Far Eastern countries provide meditation rooms as well, though I am not so sure how many travellers use such facilities.

Soon we would have to think of creating 'Rage Rooms' more than prayer rooms, not just at airports but in all public institutions, schools and colleges, parliaments and legislative assemblies. These rooms will be used for catharsis and deep psychic cleansing.

For parliaments also, it is better to have a separate room for deep catharsis and moments of deep silence, before the political leaders start their discussions and debates. Then they will not feel the need to hurl abuses and throw chairs at their opponents.

In the 1960s, Osho was the first enlightened master to anticipate this modern volatile situation of the world. As a remedy to this problem, he devised the cathartic methods of meditation, which can bring real peace to the practitioners. One such method is called 'Osho Dynamic Meditation'.

For all kinds of angry and violent people, Osho says that meditation is more helpful than anything else and dynamic meditation is particularly helpful. 'Just help the person to "cathart". He has gathered much rubbish in his heart which he has not been allowed to throw off anywhere. Help him to throw it off. Don't repress him anymore. What I call the dynamic methods of meditation can be of tremendous value to future psychiatry. Just help him to bring his madness out, whatsoever he feels like. If he wants to scream, let him.'

This meditative approach is very healthy. Almost 80 per cent of diseases are due to repressed emotions. Our heart gradually becomes weak if we keep poisoning it with repressed anger and hatred. From our childhood, we are taught to control our emotions. Nobody teaches us how to transform them.

Spiritual science teaches us to transform our emotions through catharsis and deep observation. In Osho's dynamic and other cathartic meditations, this transformation takes place. The energy is neutral and in its raw form, it can get expressed in sexuality, anger, rape and violence. The same energy, with the help of such dynamic methods, gets expressed as love, friendliness and compassion.

THE GIFT
OF THE
PRESENT

A Dangerous Man

Though so much has been written about Osho, it is difficult to describe who he was. This enlightened master spoke with astounding clarity about every aspect of human experience and consciousness.

Yet, he declared to his disciples, 'I cannot say I am a master; I can only say I am a hollow bamboo. You can make a flute out of me; existence can sing a song through me. My quality is only that I will not be in the way. I will allow existence in its purity to touch your heart.'

Osho was born on 11 December 1931 in Kuchwada, a small village in Madhya Pradesh and his parents gave him the name, Rajneesh Chandra Mohan. He died on 19 January 1990 at Osho Commune International in Pune, where his ashes are preserved in his samadhi at the Chuang Tzu Auditorium.

Osho loved books and his personal library in Pune contains about 100,000 titles. His tastes were eclectic, ranging from philosophy and religion to psychology, science, literature, history, arts, politics and poetry. All the books have been read and dated and often signed by him. Osho used a unique signature. He says, 'Thousands of times people have asked me, "What does this signature mean? Which is the language you are signing in?" It means nothing! It is no language.

My signature says nothing; it is just symbolic. It indicates something but it says nothing, it means nothing. It is not my name.'

Osho has also been criticised and condemned by priests and politicians of the world as he was not a conformist to any religion or belief system. Tom Robbins, author of *Even Cowgirls Get the Blues* and *Jitterbug Perfume*, said: 'Osho is the most dangerous man since Jesus Christ.... He's obviously a very effective man, otherwise he wouldn't be such a threat. He's saying the same things that nobody else has the courage to say.'

Guru is Like a Full Moon

A guru is the one who liberates us and for whom we have deep love, faith and reverence. A guru is a presence. Through him one gets the first glimpse of divinity. A guru creates, transforms and gives a new birth to a seeker so that with complete trust one can follow his guru while travelling through many unknown paths and doors and opening many unknown locks. His blessing is a vital phenomenon. Through a guru, we can look into our own future and can be aware of our own destiny. Through him, we start growing up like a seed trying to sprout towards the sky.

Thousands of disciples of various gurus, especially in India, celebrate Guru Purnima, the night of the full moon, to express their gratitude towards their gurus. The full moon in July is very significant and it is called Aashadh Purnima. It is such a time when we can never be sure if the full moon will be visible in the sky.

Osho has given a very poetic expression to this. He says: 'The guru is like the full moon and the disciple is like *Aashadh* (the month of clouds and rains). The moon of Sharad Purnima is beautiful because it is in the empty sky.

'If there is no disciple then, the guru is alone. If the same beauty happens in *Aashadh*, then it is something where the guru is surrounded with cloud-like disciples.

'The disciples have come with their darkness of many lives. They are like dark clouds, they are the weather of *Aashadh*. If the guru can shine like the full moon in that atmosphere of darkness, if he can produce light, only then he is the guru. That's why Aashadh Purnima is called Guru Purnima.'

This brings us to another question: Who is a guru?

In Osho's words: 'Guru means one who has gravitation, around whom you suddenly feel as if you are being pulled. The guru is a tremendous magnet with only one difference. There is a man who has charisma—you are pulled but you are pulled towards him. That is the man of charisma. He may become a great leader, a great politician. Adolf Hitler had that charisma, millions of people were pulled towards him. Then what is the difference between a charismatic leader and a guru? When you are pulled towards a guru, you suddenly feel that you are being pulled inwards, not outwards.'

When you are pulled towards Kabir, Nanak or Buddha, you have a strange feeling. The feeling of being pulled towards them and at the same time you are being pulled inwards—a very strange paradoxical phenomenon: The closer you come to your guru, the closer you come to yourself.

The more you become attracted towards the guru, the more you become independent. The more you surrender to the guru, the more you feel that you have freedom you never enjoyed before.

Guru does not exist as an ego—he exists as a pure presence and godliness radiates through him. He is transparent.

The Treasure Hunt

The world is full of poor people seeking shortcuts to get rich overnight. Every other day, we read stories of bank robberies; people are so desperate to earn a quick buck!

The other day, I came across an ancient Sufi story about one such chap. He had heard that if he went to a certain place in the desert at dawn and stood facing a distant mountain, his shadow would point to a great buried treasure. The man left his cabin before the first light of day and at dawn, stood at the designated place. His shadow shot out long and thin over the surface of the sand. 'How fortunate!' he thought as he envisioned himself with great wealth. He began digging for the treasure. He was so involved that he did not notice the sun climbing in the sky and shortening his shadow. After a while, the sun was almost half the earlier size and he cast no shadow! Overcome by worry, he started crying and thought that all his efforts went to waste since there was no sign of any treasure.

A Sufi Master who was passing by saw him and said, 'The shadow is pointing to the treasure—it's within you.'

But not all people are lucky enough to meet such a Master who can guide them towards the wealth within.

To be rich only outwardly is a waste of life. It is a sort of paralysis of our very being because getting lost in the unending, ceaseless greed for money, we become utterly hollow.

Osho says: 'Money is a way to stuff oneself with things. Money purchases everything, so it becomes important. Then you can stuff your emptiness with everything. You can have as many palaces as you want, as many cars, airplanes whatsoever you want. You can go on stuffing yourself. You are empty. An empty person is a greedy person.

'And nobody is ever fulfilled by greed. Nobody is ever fulfilled by anything because things are outside and the emptiness is inside and you cannot take things from the outside into the inside. So even if you become rich, you will remain empty.

'The inner can be fulfilled only by the inner. I am not asking you to renounce your money, that too is foolish. To continuously run after money is foolish, to renounce money is also foolish because nobody can fulfil his inner emptiness with money and nobody can fulfil it by renouncing money because both are outside. Whether you accumulate any money or renounce it, both are outside. That is not looking into the problem correctly.'

There is another related story about Mullah Nasruddin. One night, he dreamt that God had sent him a reward through an angel. The angel gave Mullah ten rupees. He felt insulted and said, 'I will take 100 rupees or I won't take anything. What a miserly approach from God!'

Still asleep, the Mullah started to shout, 'Either 100 or nothing.' And woke up with a start. He looked all around—there was nobody! He said, 'My God, I lost ninety-nine rupees unnecessarily.' He closed his eyes and apologised, 'Please come back, wherever you are. Even ninety-nine is okay, ninety-eight will do too…ninety-seven is also alright—anything will do. Just come back! Where are you?' He came down to one rupee. 'Anything from God is great. I was foolish to call God a miser. I was greedy. Forgive me. Give me just one rupee.' But the angel was gone.

The Authentic Religiousness

In *Theologia Mystica*, Osho says: 'The world is full of pseudo-religious people. If you want to know how many pseudo-religious people there are, you can count the Christians, the Mohammedans, Jains, Hindus, the Buddhists, the people who go to churches and temples and mosques and gurdwaras. These are all pseudo-religious. They have nothing to do with truth. They are believers but not religious. A religious person knows; the believer only believes. And why should one believe at all unless there are some hidden motives? Either people are afraid of hell.... They have been made afraid; their fear has been exploited for centuries. Priests became aware of the phenomenon that man lives by two things, either fear or greed. And not only priests—the politicians, pedagogues, they are all using the same strategy.

'When a child is not behaving well, you punish him. What are you doing? You are exploiting his fear. You are making him afraid that if he is going to do the same thing again he will be punished, maybe more severely. And when he behaves the way you want him to, you reward him. That is exploiting his greed. The same is the structure of all educational systems in the world: Punish and reward. The governments do it, the courts do it, teachers do it, parents do it. And the people who go to mosques and temples and churches are the people who are either afraid of hell or desiring of and greedy for heavenly pleasures.'

In the discourses on 'From Bondage to Freedom', Osho concludes: 'Religiousness is not a philosophy or a theology. It is just like love.... Religiousness is falling in love with the whole existence. And that happens when you enter within yourself and you find the lifeline running within you, joining you with all the lifelines around you, from the smallest blade of grass to the biggest star. It is one life in different manifestations, a great play of abundant energy: You have fallen in love with existence. This is religiousness.

'You don't become a Christian or a Jew or a Hindu; you simply become yourself. You are an intrinsic part of it, an organic part of it. Without you, something will be missing. That gives you a real sense of being proud. It is not ego because it is not putting yourself above others. Now you know even the smallest blade of grass is as essential as you are.

'Every man is capable of entering his own shrine and from there, can get the perspective that delivers him from all misery, suffering, tension, fear and death.

'Then each moment of his becomes a moment of ecstasy. Existence is really the only communism there is. All are equally accepted, respected, nourished. And a dance comes to your life. This dance is the transforming force.'

Finding the Right Key

The most important determinants of one's health and longevity are the personal choices made by each person. This can, of course, be frightening for those who wish to avoid taking such responsibility. But it can also be exciting for those who wish to have some control over keeping themselves healthy and happy.

Making a choice, according to Osho, means being alert about what is going on within ourselves and around us. It is evident that many of the stock answers or explanations for our being unaware are by-products of our conditioning. That's the way we avoid seeing more deeply into our own present physical and psychological state.

Osho reminds us that meditation is a way to see and accept what is happening in the present moment. By doing so, we see the truth that our current state does not encompass the whole of us. However, acknowledging the deficiencies and detriments can bring us closer to realising how and in which direction we need to grow in our awareness.

Osho has given a very simple technique for one to be in the moment. 'To be in the moment is meditation—to be here and now. One thinks neither of the past in this moment nor of the future. While being in this meditation, time stops...the world stops. The test of meditation is in the cessation of time and the inner workings of our mind. We can begin with taking smaller steps as described below:

'This is possibly the shortest meditation; it takes just about half a minute. One needs to do it at least six times a day which means giving three minutes in a whole day. But the secret is one needs to do it or act suddenly. For example, as you are walking down the street, stop suddenly—stop completely. Just freeze. For half a minute, just be present in the moment wherever you may be, in whatever condition you may be.

'Simply stop and be aware of whatever may be happening in that moment, just be alert. Then continue walking again. You may do more often than six times though not less than that. One can do this anywhere, at any time but with suddenness.'

Superconsciousness is the Goal

For years, the issue of premarital sex and live-in relationships has been discussed and debated without any conclusion and social acceptance. The issue continues to rage incessantly. The governments, the priests and the moralists have always been against any sexual freedom without marriage, while there have been powerful people—kings and royals who could live a life of freedom—and the priests and moralists would not question them. As a poet wrote: *Samarath ko nahi dosh gosain.* The powerful ones cannot be blamed. They seem to have a divine sanction. This is a clever rationalization.

For the commoners, a different code of conduct has remained in force for years. Even today, in modern society it remains the same where people are undergoing a deep psychological conditioning.

Anybody suggesting individual freedom on these issues invites criticism and condemnation, sometimes even fatwas or court cases. In spite of all this, some courageous people continue to raise this issue without fear and today it can be discussed more openly in India. Media is playing a very powerful role in this context. In March 2010, *India Today* organised a conclave and Baba Ramdev, a very popular Indian yoga teacher and Swami Satya Vedant, a well-known Osho disciple, were invited to a discussion and debate on the topic of 'Sex and Spirituality'.

Swami Satya Vedant rightly said: 'Sex is central, not god, not soul'. Few days after this conclave, on 23 March, the Supreme Court of India, gave a very significant judgement: 'Live-in, premarital sex is no offence.' The Court observed that live-in relationships between adult couples cannot be treated as offence.

'When two adult people want to live together, what is the offence? Does it amount to an offence? Living together is not an offence. It cannot be an offence', said a bench comprising Chief Justice KG Balakrishnan, Justice Deepak Verma and Justice BS Chauhan.

The Court came up with a beautiful example of an analogy from the Hindu mythology; the Court said that even Lord Krishna and Radha lived together. The apex court said there was no law which prohibits live-in relationships or premarital sex.

In 2005, a famous South Indian actress, Khushboo, in an interview to a magazine, had expressed her views on freedom of sex, allegedly endorsing premarital sex. Her views offended so many moralists that many court cases were filed against her. She had approached the apex court seeking quashing of about twenty-two criminal cases filed against her. The argument of the counsel was that her comments, allegedly endorsing premarital sex, would adversely affect the minds of young people leading to decay in moral values and ethos of the country. 'Please tell us what is the offence and under which section. Living together is a right to life,' remarked the Court apparently referring to Article 21 of the Constitution related to right to life and liberty. In 1968, Osho's discourses shook the whole country when he spoke on the topic of 'From Sex to Superconsciousness'. These talks became his first controversial book which invited large-scale criticisms and condemnations from those priests and self-appointed moralists, who had not even bothered to read the book. Osho had not preached any licentious freedom to indulge in sex but he had talked about understanding the sexual energy, befriending it and transforming it to a higher level of consciousness.

Osho says: 'It is a long way from sex to Samadhi. Samadhi is the ultimate goal, sex is only the first step. And I want to point out that those who refuse to recognise the first step, who censure the first step, cannot even reach the second step. They cannot progress at all. It is imperative to take the first step with consciousness, understanding and awareness. But be warned, sex is not an end in itself, sex is the beginning. To progress, more and more steps are required.'

Though the book, *From Sex to Superconsciousness*, has been giving a bad name to our beloved Master, it has been published in many editions, has remained a bestseller and has opened the mind of the educated members of society. It is because of these insightful discourses of Osho that now India can discuss this central issue of our life with courage.

India owes this spirit of courage and fearlessness to Osho. We must remember that the goal is not sex—free or not free—but superconsciousness.

Laugh Your Way to Self-realisation

Mullah Nasruddin is explaining the meaning of faith to his congregation. 'In the front row,' he says, 'we have Fajlu and Fajiti and their five children. Fajiti knows they are her children—that's knowledge. Fajlu believes they are his children—that is faith.'

Most of the people in the world belong to these two categories—the people of knowledge and the people of faith. Both the categories keep arguing and fighting with each other. Then there is a third category—a real minority, they are the wise ones who do not take a position of knowledge or faith. They say: 'We do not know, so there is no question of believing or not believing.' They consider themselves mere observers or watchers. They laugh at the ridiculousness of arrogance of knowledge and blindness of belief. This category of wise people is regarded as the category of idiots by the other two categories. The wise ones accept it and do not take life so seriously and they laugh at the whole situation. They do not laugh at others as it might hurt them. Rather they laugh at themselves and their laughter makes them religious in the true sense.

Mullah Nasruddin was one such religious person who could always laugh at himself. World needs such non-serious people today as it has become too serious. This heaviness of seriousness leads to violence. A non-serious person is full of zest and humour and he laughs at himself and his follies and also makes other people's life lighter. His laughter is infectious.

Osho says: 'The sense of humour should be directed towards oneself—it is a very great thing to laugh at oneself and he who can laugh at himself gradually becomes full of concern and compassion for others. In the entire world no event, no subject, invites laughter like oneself.'

Laughing at oneself can lead to self-realisation. It happens when we do not cling to the fiction of our ego. And nothing kills ego as effectively as laughter does. In the moments of hearty laughter, the ego disappears just like dewdrops disappear in the morning sun.

Intuition is More Powerful than Intellect

My intuition says that Steve Jobs will be born again, this time in India and become a sannyasin. He was a great man of science but deep within his being, he was a man of meditation and intuition. In his last birth, he might have travelled to India and was touched by the Eastern mysticism deeply. This may have become his unfulfilled desire and a reason to be born in India, to experience it totally. Also, it is very much possible that in his next birth, he may achieve the same depth in meditation as the height he achieved in technology in his previous birth.

Steven Paul Jobs was a rare genius. He had a wonderful combination of brilliance of the Western mind and mystical dimension of the Eastern heart. He was born in San Francisco, California on 24 February 1955. His biological parents, unwed college graduates, Joanne Schieble and Abdulfattah Jandali, had him adopted by a lower middle-class couple from south of the Bay Area, Paul and Clara Jobs. He attended college for only six months after which he dropped out. It is reported that he spent a lot of time learning about Eastern mysticism and adopted strange diets, fasting or eating only fruits. Those were the days of the hippies and he also enjoyed being a hippie for some time. He even travelled to India with a friend to seek enlightenment at the age of nineteen.

His biography tells us about his India sojourn in the summer of 1974. It reveals some details about his experiences in India during a seven-month trip and how he learnt about the power of intuition in this country.

'The people in the Indian countryside don't use their intellect like we do, they use their intuition instead, and their intuition is far more developed than the rest of the world. Intuition is a very powerful thing, more powerful than intellect, in my opinion. That's had a big impact on my work,' Jobs later recalled to Walter Isaacson, the biographer.

Jobs goes on to say that Western rational thought is not an innate human characteristic but is learned. 'In the villages of India, they never learned it. They learned something else, which is in some ways just as valuable but in other ways, is not. That is the power of intuition and experiential wisdom,' he said.

Jobs's intuitive understanding reminds me of the wisdom of Kabir, the mystic saint of India, who ridiculed the bookish knowledge of pundits and taught the importance of experiencing the truth with oneself: *Likha likhi ki hai nahi, dekha dekhi baat.* One cannot find truth in scriptures—one can only discover it experiencing it within. This experiencing is what we call intuition.

Osho defines the word intuition. He says: 'You know the other word, "tuition". Tuition means somebody else is giving it to you. Intuition means nobody is giving it to you, it is growing within yourself. And because it is not given to you by somebody else, it cannot be put into words.'

He adds: 'Intuition can give you answers for ultimate questions—not verbally but existentially. You need not ask, what is truth? Instinct won't hear, it is deaf. Intellect will hear but it can only philosophise, it is blind, it can't see. Intuition is a seer, it has eyes. It sees the truth—there is no question of thinking about it.

Instinct and intuition are both independent of you. Instinct is in the power of nature, of unconscious nature and intuition is in the hands of the superconscious universe, the consciousness that surrounds the whole universe, the oceanic consciousness of which we are just small islands or better, icebergs because we can melt into it and become one with it.'

Steve Jobs says his seven-month stay in Indian villages made him 'see the craziness' of the Western world as well as its capacity for rational thought.

'If you just sit and observe, you will see how restless your mind is. If you try to calm it, it will only make it worse. But over time it does calm and when it does, there's room to hear more subtle things—that's when your intuition starts to blossom,' he says.

This is the right observation and perfect beginning for the inner journey of meditation.

Not by Bread Alone

We Indians boast of our country being highly spiritual. But an honest look into our lives will reveal that we are perhaps the most materialistic people in the world. We may go to temples, regularly do our prayers, yet, our prayers are usually to ask for favours from our gods: More money, marriage of our children or good health.

We need to understand our priorities of needs. Osho points out: 'First, the bodily needs have to be fulfilled. If they are not fulfilled, you will not have higher needs arising. A hungry person cannot think of music.'

Similarly, when Swami Vivekananda was asked in the United States, 'Why have you come here to teach?' he replied, 'Here I can talk about Vedanta, the ultimate truth. But in India, seeing people hungry, I feel ashamed of talking about God. It is insulting to those poor people.'

Osho also reminds us what Jesus said, 'Man cannot live by bread alone' but adds that 'if your body is ill, hungry, in pain, you cannot compose poetry, you cannot paint. Even if you paint, your painting will remain that of suffering. If you write poetry, it will be nothing but slogans. The bodily needs have to be fulfilled first. Yes, don't get stuck there.'

We need to remember that we have to go beyond the body but we cannot bypass it. Yes, we need to know the joys of the mind, the beauties of the mind, art, poetry, painting, music; great joys of the mind. When they are fulfilled, we move to the third level of needs, those of the soul. Then meditation becomes important. Osho says: 'Only a person who has lived deeply in music is capable of meditation because music prepares the background, creates the space, the context, in which meditation becomes simple. And the person whose soul-needs are fulfilled, whose meditation-needs are fulfilled, will be able to pray.'

Prayer thus, is not to ask for material favours but is the fragrance of the flower of meditation. Prayer is the ultimate.

Meditation Awakens

There are two ways of living our life—consciously or unconsciously, either mechanically, robot-like or with full awareness. Most people live their life as if they are half-asleep, they act semiconsciously. That is why we see so much misery and anguish around us. People simply react unconsciously or mechanically. Someone calls us names or insults us and we become furious and want to kill him. This behaviour cannot be called a conscious or meditative behaviour.

This is mechanical. It creates a chain reaction in all of us and we become chained. This is bondage, not freedom.

Meditation is a science, the pure science of awareness—to be free. Meditation is freedom. It is watchfulness, witnessing each act that we do. It is an alchemical process to bring metamorphosis within ourselves. It is a revolution in the individual and finally, a revolution in the society.

One awakened being who goes through this revolution becomes a Buddha, the enlightened one, who shows light to millions of people for thousands of years. It is the magic of meditation. What even one Buddha can do is incomparable. Thousands of social reformers are not capable of doing that. Social reformers bring changes only superficially, the cosmetic reforms, but Buddhas bring transformations deep within.

Science is something universal—that which is applicable to all while belief systems are not universal, they are local or parochial in nature. You can argue or fight about them. They lead us nowhere. They do not lead to self-realisation. Meditation, on the other hand, is an inward journey, the unknown treasures that we carry within us, the joy and bliss that are within us. A blissful person, an illumined person brings joy and light to others. He is a blessing, a benediction.

Osho observes: 'Meditation is observation, looking in. You need not have a belief system as a prerequisite. An atheist can meditate, just as anybody else can because meditation is only a method of turning inwards.'

Monk and the Zorba

A new disciple had a question for Osho: 'Sometimes when you speak, I get the vision of living a kind of Zorba the Greek life—lusty and passionate—and I think this is the way. At other times, I feel you are saying that the way is to sit silently, watchful, dispassionate, cool and calm like a monk. So, who are we to be—Zorbas or monks?'

Osho responded, 'I am trying to create Zorba the Buddha.' He said: 'Eat, drink and being merry is perfectly good in itself: Nothing is wrong in it. But it is not enough. Soon you will get tired of it. One cannot just go on eating, drinking and "merrying". Soon the merry-go-round turns into a sorry-go-round. Yet, Zorba the Greek is the very foundation of Zorba, the Buddha. Buddha arises out of that experience. Live in this world because this world gives ripening, maturity and integrity. The challenges of this world give you a centring, an awareness. That awareness becomes the ladder. Then you can move from Zorba to Buddha.'

Health and Wholeness
Lie Beyond Duality

Zen master Sosan says cryptically: 'The great way is not difficult for those who have no preferences.'

It is difficult for us to comprehend that one could live without preferences. Yet, it is already the case with nature—trees, birds, animals, rivers, mountains, planets are all moving with the natural flow of existence without any preference. It is only man who finds this difficult. And the difficulty comes from his mind.

Mind is a great divider, an arbitrator of good and bad, right and wrong. Give your mind anything and soon you will see that it has created a duality. First, it divides everything and then it creates conflicts between the divided parts. Then, in a vicious circle, it tries to give solutions to the conflicts created by it. It is like disease giving us the cure, telling us ways to health.

Contrasting the Eastern and the Western approaches, Osho explains: 'The West says mind can become ill and can be healthy. Western psychology depends on this. But for the East, mind as such is the disease, it cannot be healthy. The word "health" is beautiful. Health, healing, whole, holy—they all come from the same root.'

All the sages of the East have advised us to meditate and

transcend the mind to be in the realm of witnessing consciousness. Krishna and Ashtavakra term it as *sakshi bhav*, J Krishnamurti calls it choiceless awareness.

Mind is a phenomenon of choice. Osho proclaims: 'You choose and you are in misery. Choose and you are in the trap because whenever you choose, you have chosen something against something else. If you are for something, you must be against something: You cannot be only for, you cannot be only against. When the "for" enters, the "against" follows as a shadow. When you choose, you divide. Then you say, "This is right, this is wrong."

'But life is a unity. Existence remains undivided, existence remains in a deep unison. This is natural *Advaita*, non-duality, the real health that comes from oneness and wholeness.'

Hello, Happiness

I have seen and known people who wake up every morning complaining about life. I do not know why. There seems to be no apparent reason. Perhaps they did not sleep well the night before or had nightmares during their sleep. Perhaps they are afraid that they will have to do a lot of work after getting out of their bed. Or they feel that they are being forced to face something unpleasant, something they cannot escape and that is why they feel miserable.

When the day begins this way, it is going to be this way the whole day and the following night is also going to be full of unease. And the same will happen next morning. The undercurrent of unhappiness will continue whatever one does. This then becomes a vicious circle of unending misery.

As I see it, we ourselves are responsible for this sorry state of affairs. We cannot blame others. Blaming others is very unintelligent and childish. It is not going to bring any joy to our lives. It will create even more helplessness and despair.

Stephen Hawking says, 'People won't have time for you if you are always angry and complaining.'

Then what is the solution? How can we be happy?

I have found a simple answer in a Sufi story.

It is a story of a Sufi mystic Abdulla, who was never seen

unhappy in his whole life. He was always playful and laughing. He gave this message to everybody who came to him—not through words but by example. His happiness and laughter was infectious. In his last days, when he was about to die, he was laughing the same way he laughed always. This was a matter of surprise to all his disciples and one of them finally asked him: 'Beloved Master, we cannot believe that you can be happy and laughing even now when you are on your deathbed. We are feeling sad and miserable. We always wanted to ask you many times in your life why you are never sad. How did you manage to be happy in life? How are you managing it now as well at the time of your death?'

The Sufi master replied: 'It is simple. If you know how to remain happy in life, you will not have to worry when you die. When I was a young man, I used to be a really miserable person. But then I met my enlightened master. My master looked to me always happy, sitting under a tree and laughing for no reason at all. I wondered that he had nothing, nobody to take care of him and still he was happy. I asked him, "Master, I cannot believe that you can be happy and laughing just sitting under this tree. What is your secret?"

'The old man said, "One day I was also as sad and miserable as you are. I meditated deeply and then it dawned on me: You are unhappy because you choose to be unhappy. The same way, you can choose to be happy. Whatever is happening in your life is your own choice."

'Since that day, I have been very decisive. Every morning when I wake up, I say to myself, Abdulla, what do you want today—happiness or misery? What do you prefer today? Then it becomes simple—I simply choose to be happy. This is my daily meditation.'

Osho enlightens us to take hold of our own life. 'Just look the whole existence is celebrating. The trees are not serious, the birds are not serious. The rivers and oceans are wild and everywhere there is fun, everywhere there is joy and delight. Watch existence, listen to the existence and become part of it.'

Osho says that once you have started seeing the beauty of life, ugliness starts disappearing. If you start looking at life with joy, sadness starts disappearing. You cannot have heaven and hell together, you can have only one. It is your choice.

OSHO

AN

INVITATION

Osho——an Invitation

The journey of self-realisation begins with the help of a master who has already attained his ultimate potential, his illumination; who is no more his ego and has become a vehicle of the divine. He radiates godliness.

The illumination of the master becomes an invitation to the unlit lamp of the disciple who gropes in the dark looking for somebody who can show him the way. To find such a master is really a blessing, a benediction. Half the inner journey is over by meeting such a master and the other half is over when the disciples come to fruition and become masters themselves. Somebody asked Osho: 'Who are you?'

Osho replied: 'I am an invitation. I am an invitation for all those who are seeking, searching and have a deep longing in their hearts to find their home.'

A true enlightened master is an open invitation to one and all, without any discrimination of caste, colour or creed. He invites everybody to come and drink from the river of his wisdom, love and compassion and quench their thirst to seek the truth. Just as a river does not discriminate between deserving and the undeserving ones, it shares its water with everybody without asking anything in return. A river simply flows and so does the enlightened master, who has become one with the infinite source of life. By sharing his light the master does not lose anything, rather it becomes manifold. And when his disciples also become illumined, it proves the true enlightenment of the master. The Bauls of Bengal go on singing, 'Come Beloved, come.' They go on sending their invitations. Love is nothing but an opening, a receptivity, a welcome, an invitation, that I am ready; come, please.

There is a beautiful statement of Mawlana Jalaluddin Rumi, one of the greatest Sufi masters ever.

> *Come, come, whoever you are;*
> *wanderer, worshipper, lover of learning...*
> *It does not matter.*
> *Ours is not a caravan of despair.*
> *Come, even if you have broken your vow*
> *a thousand times.*
> *Come, come, yet again come.*

'Come, come, whoever you are...sinner, unconscious, living a life which is not glorious, divine, meaningful; living a life which has no poetry, no joy, a life of hell.... Whosoever you are,' Mawlana says, 'come, I am ready to receive you. Be my guest!'

The master is a host; he refuses nobody. True masters never refuse anybody. They cannot. If they start refusing people, then there is no hope. If you go under a tree, a shady tree—tired of your journey and the burning sun on your head—and the tree refuses you, it does not give you refuge, it does not shelter you? This never happens. The tree is always ready to give you shelter, its shadow, its fruits, its flowers and its fragrance.

Never Born Never Died

Osho never wrote his biography. The disciples did ask him several times why he hadn't written one. His answer is really incredible: 'All autobiographies are ego-biographies. It is not the story of the soul. As long as you do not know what soul is, whatever you write is ego-biography'.

Neither Jesus, nor Krishna, nor Buddha have written their autobiographies. Writing or speaking about oneself has not been possible for those who have known themselves, because after knowing, the person changes into something so formless that what we call the facts of his life—facts like his date of birth, events, all dissolve. They cease to have meaning. The awakening of a soul is so cataclysmic that after it occurs, when you open your eyes you find that everything is lost. Once you know your soul, an autobiography is only a dreamlike version of oneself, like writing an account of your dreams. Such writing has no more value than a fantasy, a fairy tale. So it is difficult for an awakened person to write. On becoming awakened and aware, he finds that there is nothing worth writing. It was all a dream. The experience of becoming aware remains, but what is known through the experience cannot be written down.

Reducing such an experience to words makes it seem insipid

and absurd. A dying Buddha was asked: 'Where will you go after death?' He said, 'I have been nowhere, so where can I go after death?'

The meaning of Buddha-hood is 'nowhereness'. One is nowhere, so the question of being somewhere does not arise. If you can be quiet and silent, only breathing remains like the air inside a bubble.

When there are no thoughts there is nothing but breathing. So Buddha says, 'I was only a bubble. Where was I? A bubble has burst and you are asking where it has gone.'

Autobiography does not survive. Deeply speaking, the soul itself does not survive. So far we understand only that the ego does not survive. For thousands of years, we have been told that the ego does not survive when one attains self-knowledge.

But to put it correctly, the soul itself does not survive. Buddha said, 'The soul also does not survive; we become non-soul.' Mahavira talked only of the death of the ego; that much could be understood.

It is not that Mahavira did not know that even the soul does not survive, but he had in mind our limited understanding. Therefore, he spoke only of giving up the ego, knowing that the soul would automatically dissolve.

The idea of the soul is a projection of the ego. But Buddha revealed the secret which had been closely guarded for so long. That created difficulties. If the soul does not survive either, they said, then everything is useless.

Where are we? Buddha was right. Everything is like a dream sequence, like the rainbow colours formed on a bubble. The colours die when the bubble bursts.

The Male Ego Conflicts

The relationship between a male and his father is often full of conflict. According to a study by California State University-Fullerton, men who had positive childhood relationships with their fathers are more able to handle stress and emotional distress later in life than those that didn't. Unfortunately, not every male enjoys a nurturing, positive relationship with his father. There are a variety of reasons why some fathers and sons don't get along.

Osho talks about a Great Russian novelist, Turgenev, who has written a book—perhaps his best, his masterpiece—*Fathers and Sons*. The book is about the struggle between the fathers and the sons, because the fathers would like the sons to be their replicas. Naturally, they will not allow the sons any freedom. Obedience they expect; they expect their sons to be their carbon copies.

He says in this book that the relationship between a father and son is always one of conflict. There is no other tie, except the tie of conflict between them. The son is the rightful successor of the father and therefore, is always engaged in removing him. He waits eagerly for him to vacate his position. The son hates the dominance of the father in most of the family affairs. When this becomes intolerable or unbearable for the son, he can even go to the extent of killing his father in anger. This conflict is an eternal one and a chapter was added to this hate-saga in the shape of royal killings in Nepal in 2001.

If we look at this situation in psychological terms, we come across some startling revelations.

Freud did lot of research on this subject. He said that people worship God as father because some time in the beginning they must have killed some dominant father, somebody who was too dictatorial. It is a well-known fact that many a king have been killed by their sons because the king lived on, thus making the heir wait endlessly. The son was gaining age and it seemed that he was not going to live to be a king; the only possibility lay in the death of the father. Many kings have imprisoned their fathers and taken over the throne, because they saw that there seemed to be no possibility of his natural death—at least while there was time to enjoy being a king! What would be the point when you are seventy-five or eighty when your father dies and you succeed? Within a year or two you would be gone too.

Osho appreciates the psychological insights of Sigmund Freud who says that because somewhere in the past man had to kill the father he felt the guilt of what he had done. And out of that guilt he started worshipping the ancestors, the fathers, the elderly people, old people. All this respect has arisen out of a guilt that is deep-set in the human heart. Man started inventing a God as father, raising temples in his memory, statues, priests praying, worshippers worshipping. Behind this whole scene and drama of religion, Sigmund Freud finds only one single fact and that is: Somewhere in the past man has behaved so badly with his father—perhaps murdered—that he cannot forgive him. So the only way is to pray, make God your father, the creator of the world. All these hypotheses...it was a very original insight.

Lao Tzu says: 'The more you try to make sons listen to their fathers, the more they will go against their fathers'. And Lao Tzu has been proved correct. In the last 5,000 years, man has tried to make the son obedient to the father and the result is an increasing abyss between the two. A son touches his father's feet and calculates what he will inherit from him. It is said that the sons of rich fathers never lament the father's death. They cannot. Perhaps they are happy. The sons of kings have been known to bring about the death of their fathers. All around us there are manipulations and calculations.

There is no inner necessity that the son should agree with the father. In fact it seems far better that he should not agree. That's how evolution happens. If every child agrees with the father then there will be no evolution, because the father will agree with his own father, so everybody will be where God left Adam and Eve—naked, outside the gate of the Garden of Eden. Everybody will be there. Because sons have disagreed with their fathers, forefathers, with their whole tradition, man has evolved.

This whole evolution is a tremendous disagreement with the past.

The Green-eyed Monster: Jealousy

Someone on the internet defines jealousy as: 'An emotion experienced by one who perceives that another person is giving something that s/he wants (typically attention, love, or affection) to a third party. For example, a child will likely become jealous when her parent gives sweets to a sibling but not to her. On an interpersonal level it is a threat felt from an outsider to an important relationship in which one is involved and produces feelings of anger and fear. It is a state of fear, suspicion or envy over one's possessions.'

This is just one aspect of jealousy—there are several other aspects of this emotion also that we suffer from in our daily life. A man becomes immediately jealous when another man attracts his woman—and the same is the case with woman also. This does not happen only to ordinary men or women, this happens to all, and even to those rare scientists who are able to reveal the deepest mysteries of the universe, and to those great thinkers and philosophers who reveal to us the greatest mysteries of our mind. It happens to everyone who is human.

Here I would like to quote what scientists have discovered recently (courtesy *Daily Mail*): 'Scientists discover the jealousy lobe: The green-eyed monster that lives in your brain. It is a vice that few can avoid but that nobody craves. Now the area of the brain which controls jealousy has been found, scientists have announced. It is the same part which detects real physical pain—perhaps explaining why feeling envious of your lover's philandering ways hurts so much. The spot which makes people delight in others' misfortune—called schadenfreude—was also located by the team.

'It's interesting the part of the brain which detects physical pain is also associated with mental pain,' said Hidehiko Takahashi, who led the research. 'Assessing these feelings of jealousy will possibly be helpful in mental care such as counseling.'

'Envy is corrosive and ugly, and it can ruin your life,' Richard Smith, a professor of psychology at the University of Kentucky told *The New York Times*. 'If you're an envious person, you have a hard time appreciating a lot of the good things that are out there, because you're too busy worrying about how they reflect on the self.'

In the experiments, nineteen students were asked to talk of a more successful rival while having MRI scans, which monitor brain activity. A part of their frontal lobe became more active when the students felt jealous of their rivals, the Japanese study showed. They then read a story in which the subject of their envy suffered a series of misfortunes, including food poisoning. Their scan data showed the mishaps sparked greater activity in the 'reward reaction' part of the brain, which normally lights up when receiving social and financial fortune. 'We have a saying in Japanese, "The misfortunes of others are the taste of honey,"' said Mr Takahashi. 'The ventral striatum is processing that "honey."'

And there appears to be a relationship between jealousy and schadenfreude. The scientists noted that the more jealous one person was of another, the more schadenfreude they felt at that person's downfall.

'We now have a better understanding of the mechanism at work when people take pleasure in another's misfortune,' said Mr Takahashi.

'This is the way other needs-processing systems like hunger and thirst work,' Matthew Lieberman of the psychology department at the University of California, Los Angeles, who co-wrote a commentary that accompanies the report, told *The New York Times*.

'The hungrier or thirstier that you feel, the more pleasurable it is when you finally eat or drink.'

There's so much to write on this subject that one would need thousands of pages. But if we just remember one point, we won't need thousands of pages to understand—and that point is jealousy is there because love is missing:

Osho points out: 'Love is the ultimate law. You just have to discover its beauties, its treasures. You have not to repeat, parrot-like, all the great values which make man the highest expression of consciousness on this planet. You should exercise them in your relationship.

'And this has been my strange experience: If one partner starts moving on the right lines, the other follows sooner or later. Because they both are hungry for love, but they don't know how to approach it.'

No university teaches that love is an art and that life is not already given to you; that you have to learn from scratch.

And it is good that we have to discover by our own hands every treasure that is hidden in life...and love is one of the greatest treasures in existence.

But instead of becoming fellow travellers in search of love, beauty and truth, people are wasting their time in fighting, in jealousy.

Just become a little alert and start the change from your side—don't expect it from the other side. It will begin from the other side too. And it costs nothing to smile, it costs nothing to love, it costs nothing to share your happiness with somebody you love.

Meditation: A Quantum Leap of Awareness

With so many gurus around these days teaching and preaching, millions of people have heard about meditation. But I am not so sure if they can really meditate or relax into their being. In the past, meditation may have been easy as people used to live a simple life. Now it is not that easy. One cannot just sit in meditation—just sitting, doing nothing, thinking nothing, is not possible for the modern man. The mind goes on spinning all kinds of strange ideas and stories, one can witness all the horror films in one's mind without going to a movie theatre. This creates uneasiness for the body also, so the body cannot be still. In such a situation, one should simply forget about the soul. One is not going to experience it. One needs to relax first—physically and mentally—to realise one's soul or consciousness.

After experimenting with thousands of people in meditation camps, Osho has an insight to share: 'To begin with relaxation is difficult; hence, in the East we have never started from relaxation. But if you want to, I have a certain idea how you should start.... While I was taking camps of meditators I used a gibberish meditation and the Kundalini meditation. If you want to start from relaxation, then these meditations have to be done first. They will take out all tensions from your mind and body, and then relaxation is very easy. You don't know how much you are holding in, and that is the cause of tension.

'The gibberish meditation was that everybody was allowed to say loudly whatever comes into his mind. And it was such a joy to hear what people were saying, irrelevant, absurd—because I was the only witness. People were doing all kinds of things, and the only condition was that you should not touch anybody else. You could do whatever you wanted....

'One man used to sit every day in front—he must have been a broker or something—and as the meditation would begin, first he would smile, just at the idea of what he was going to do. Then he would take up his phone, "Hello, hello..." From the corner of his eyes he would go on looking at me. I would avoid looking at him so as not to disturb his meditation. He was selling his shares, purchasing—the whole hour he was on the phone.

'Everybody was doing the strange things that they were holding back. When the meditation would end there were ten minutes for relaxation and you could see that in those ten minutes people fell down—not with any effort, but because they were utterly tired. All the rubbish had been thrown out, so they had a certain cleanliness, and they relaxed. Thousands of people...and you could not even think that there were a thousand people.'

Osho adds: 'People used to come to me and say, "Prolong those ten minutes, because in our whole life we have never seen such relaxation, such joy. We had never thought we would ever understand what awareness is, but we felt it was coming."

'So if you want to start with relaxation, first you have to go through a cathartic process. Dynamic meditation, Latihan, kundalini or gibberish. You may not know from where this word gibberish comes; it comes from a Sufi mystic whose name was Jabbar—and that was his only meditation. Whoever would come, he would say, "Sit down and start"—and people knew what he meant. He never talked, he never gave any discourses; he simply taught people gibberish.

'For example, once in a while he would give people a demonstration. For half an hour he would talk all kinds of nonsense in nobody knows what language. It was not a language; he would go on teaching people just whatever came to his mind. That was his only teaching—and to those who had understood it he would simply say, "Sit down and start."

'But Jabbar helped many people to become utterly silent. How long you can go on?—the mind becomes empty. Slowly, slowly a deep nothingness...and in that nothingness a flame of awareness. It is always present, surrounded by your gibberish. The gibberish has to be taken out; that is your poison.

'The same is true about the body. Your body has tensions. Just start making any movements that the body wants to make. You should not manipulate it. If it wants to dance, it wants to jog, it wants to run, it wants to roll down on the ground, you should not do it, you should simply allow it. Tell the body, "You are free, do whatever you want"—and you will be surprised, "My God. All these things the body wanted to do but I was holding back, and that was the tension."

'So there are two kinds of tension, the body tensions and the mind tensions. Both have to be released before you can start relaxation, which will bring you to awareness. But beginning from awareness is far easier, and particularly for those who can understand the process of awareness, which is very simple. The whole day you are using it about things—cars, in the traffic—even in the traffic you survive! It is absolutely mad.... You are using awareness without being aware of it, but only about outside things. It is the same awareness that has to be used for the inside traffic. When you close your eyes there is a traffic of thoughts, emotions, dreams, imaginations; all kinds of things start flashing by.... And slowly, slowly, as awareness grows your whole personality starts changing. From unawareness to awareness is the greatest quantum leap.'

The Spiritual Friendship

Every year on 5 August, people celebrate World Friendship Day. Friends are encouraged to express their beautiful feelings of friendship through messages on mobile phones and on electronic mail. Individually I find that my life is full of friends and I feel really really rich.

It is beautiful to feel that you have friends in the world. This feeling must be nourished and nurtured in every possible way. The world media can do this very effectively if it highlights such news more than the bad news that vitiates our life. We are already being burdened by enormous madness and misery created by the politicians in the world! There are storms and storms of greed, lust, anger, violence, torture and terrorism. It is becoming very difficult to protect a small burning lamp of friendship and love in such storms.

Gautama the Buddha had declared that he would come to the world again as a Friend after twenty-five centuries, perhaps he could foresee what was going to be needed today. Osho created his commune of brotherhood of the citizens of the whole world called commune—a meeting place for friends. He declared himself a *Kalyanmitra*—a Benevolent Friend.

We—his disciples, lovers and friends—must remember this and keep reminding each other. We must protect this tiny lamp of love.

This should be our prime concern and meditation. Our life is worth living only when it is throbbing and pulsating in the cool breeze of friendship. Be welcoming and grateful to it but first one needs to learn the art of being friendly to oneself. You cannot be friendly to others if you are not friendly to yourself first.

In the *Dhammapada, the Way of the Buddha*, Osho makes a clear statement and gives a perspective about friendship and love: 'Making friends with the idea of using people is taking a wrong step from the very beginning. Friendship has to be a sharing. If you have something, share it—and whosoever is ready to share with you is a friend. It is not a question of need. It is not a question that when you are in danger a friend has to come to your aid. That is irrelevant—he may come, he may not come, but if he doesn't come, it is perfectly okay. It is his decision to come or not to come. You don't want to manipulate him; you don't want to make him feel guilty. You will not have any grudge. You will not say to him, "When I was in need you didn't turn up—what kind of friend are you?"

'Friendship is not something of the marketplace. Friendship is one of those rare things which belong to the temple and not to the shop. But you are not aware of that kind of friendship; you will have to learn it. Friendship is great art. Love has natural instincts behind it; friendship has no natural instincts behind it. Friendship is something conscious; love is unconscious.

'What we call love is more animalistic than human. Friendship is absolutely human. It has something for which there is no inbuilt mechanism in your biology; it is non-biological. Hence one rises in friendship; one does not fall in friendship. It has a spiritual dimension.

'There is no need to think for the whole future. Think in terms of the moment and present. Live in the present. If this moment is full of friendship and the fragrance of friendship, why be worried about the next moment. It is bound to be of higher, deeper quality. It will bring the same fragrance to the higher altitude.

There is no need to think about it—just live the moment in deep friendship.

'Friendship need not be addressed to anyone in particular; that is also a rotten idea—that you have to be friends with certain person. Just be friendly. Rather than creating friendship create friendliness. Let it become a quality of your being, a climate that surrounds you, so you are friendly with whomsoever you come in contact.

'This whole existence has to be befriended! And if you can befriend existence, existence will befriend you a thousandfold. It returns to you in the same coin, but multiplied. It echoes you that my world was full of friendship and really rich...'

The Infinite Beauty of Sannyas

Do not go to the garden of flowers!
O Friend! Go not there;
In your body is the garden of flowers.
Take your seat on the thousand petals of the lotus,
and there gaze on the Infinite Beauty.

Thus says saint Kabir, the mystic of paradox.

This is what exactly is sannyas—an inner flower, a lotus, blossoming in meditation. Meditation is the soul of sannyas and fragrance of love its expression.

For thousands of years, the East, specially India, has known sannyas. You could say that there's nothing new about sannyas. Yes, there's nothing new, but there's something eternal and undying about sannyas. Each time an enlightened mystic appears on the earth, he gives new life to sannyas. There was sannyas in the Upanishadic time and Krishna's time and it was very life—affirmative and playful. Then there was sannyas in Buddha's time and Mahavira's time, and Adi Shankara's time when sannyas took a new turn towards renunciation. Again there was a great revolution in sannyas with the arrival of saints like Kabir and Guru Nanak: Sannyasis could come back to the world and stay in the thick of the world. Kabir himself continued working as a *julaha*, a weaver, and kept singing his divine songs to raise the consciousness of people. Guru Nanak liberated people from all kinds of hypocrisies and pretensions prevalent in the name of sannyas.

Sannyas reached its climax, an ultimate glory and dignity when Osho opened its doors to all by introducing it in the most radical form—with meditation in the marketplace, and embracing life in all its colours. Osho gave it a rebirth as Neo-Sannyas.

In *The Perennial Path: The Art of Living*, Osho says: 'The sannyas, like love, cannot become an institution. Institutions are made for security. Sannyas is a personal experience, like love it blooms and spreads. In an institution it is devoid of all its beauty, interest and mystery. An institution becomes like a prison for the sannyasi if he cannot return to the samsara if he so desires. But the state of sannyas is one's personal decision, one has the freedom to experience it fully and courageously and without any regrets. I know hundreds of sannyasis who are miserable because they cannot return to the samsara. I wish to emphasise on this state of the sannyas. Just as science is the gift of the West to the world, sannyas is the great gift from the East, along with the greatest individuals of Asia like Buddha, Mahavira, Christ and Muhammed.'

And in another discourse, he talks about phony sannyas: 'The phony sannyas is escapist. It teaches you not to enjoy life, it teaches you not to love music, it teaches you not to cherish beauty. It teaches you to destroy all the sources that beautify your existence. It teaches you to escape to the caves, ugly caves, to turn your back towards the world that God has given as a gift to you.

'The phony sannyas is not only against the world, it is against God too, because to be against the world is to be against the creator of the world. If you hate the painting you are bound to hate the painter. If you dislike the dance, how can you like the dancer? God is the painter, the world is his painting. God is the musician, the world is his music. God is the dancer, Nataraj, and the world is his dance. If you renounce the world, indirectly you are renouncing God.'

He concludes: 'The sannyas that teaches you how to live in the world and yet float above it like a lotus flower, like a lotus leaf, remaining in the water and yet untouched by the water, remaining in the world and yet not allowing the world to enter into you, being in the world yet not being of the world, that is true renunciation.'

Osho invites the people of the whole world to meditate being in the world and celebrate their life, making this world a more beautiful place to live in. A sannyasin can change the very atmosphere around him by transforming himself with meditation and by sharing his love with others. And to him, meditation is not something serious, not holier-than-thou crap. It is playful. It is fun!

Synthesis That Produces a
Beautiful Organic Unity

Once Osho was asked: 'Is it right to say that movements in the West like Arica, Zen, Sufism, EST and TM are the inevitable synthesis of Eastern mysticism and Western science?'

Osho replied: 'East and West are polarities. If you try to synthesise them—take something of the East and something of the West and make a hotchpotch out of it—it will be a compromise, not a synthesis.

'It will be mechanical, not organic. You can put things together—that is a mechanical unity—but you cannot put a tree together, you cannot put a human being together. The unity of a tree grows, it comes from its innermost core and it spreads towards its circumference. It arises in the centre.

'A mechanical unity can be put together from the outside: You can put a car or a clock together but they have neither centre nor soul. It is a unity put together from the outside. It works; it is utilitarian. But a tree, a bird, a human—you cannot put them together. They grow. Their unity comes from their innermost core. They have a centre.

'A compromise is a mechanical unity: A synthesis is an

organic growth. So whatever is happening in the name of EST, TM or Arica, is mechanical unity.

'The greatest danger is this: The East has developed great insight into religion and the West, great insight into science. When a person from the West starts searching in the East, his attitude is scientific. He can understand only that which is scientific in the East. Eastern science is rudimentary. When a religious person from the East goes to the West he looks into Western religion which is very rudimentary. And he can understand only religious language.

'Now what is happening? East and West are meeting in Arica, EST, TM, and other so-called spiritual movements, and just the opposite of what was expected is happening.

'It is not Eastern religion meeting Western science, it is Eastern science meeting Western religion.'

Osho warns against creating a synthesis of the religions of the world. He says: 'Read the Koran, the Vedas, the Bible, the Dhammapada, find similarities but the Koran is beautiful only because of those things which are not in the Gita.'

Beauty is in uniqueness; similarities become clichés, they become meaningless and monotonous. The Himalayas are beautiful because they have something unique that is not in the Alps. And the Ganga is beautiful because it has something that is not in the Amazon. Of course, both are rivers; there are many similarities, but if you keep looking for similarities you will live in a boring world.

Osho concludes: 'Go into your innermost being. If you go beyond the object, you have gone beyond the West; if you go beyond the subject, you have gone beyond the East.

'Then the transcendental arises; the synthesis is there. When it has happened within you, you can spread it without also. The synthesis has to happen within human beings, not in books, dissertations, PhD theses. An organic unity is possible only in an organic way.'

Forget the others,
Realise Your Self

The disciples from around the world asked Osho about all the practical problems they were facing in their daily life—such as jealousy or greed—and Osho explained in very simple language that everybody could understand.

About Jealousy: 'It means ego, it means unconsciousness. It means that you have not known even a moment of joy and bliss; you are living in misery. Jealousy is a by-product of misery, ego, unconsciousness. And not only about jealousy, remember, about all problems—greed....'

Somebody says, 'I am very greedy about money. How can I get rid of this greed for money?'

Osho explains: 'It is not a question of money. Greed is greed. If you get rid of money you will become greedy for God; greed will still be there. The night Jesus was saying goodbye to his disciples, one of the disciples asked him, "Lord, you are leaving us. There is one question, and it is on the minds of all your disciples. In the kingdom of God you will be sitting at the right side of God himself—obviously, you will be his right hand. And who will be sitting next to you? Amongst us twelve, who will be the second to you? That is the most important thing in our heads. Please say something about it; otherwise, once you are gone it will be impossible for us to decide and we will be quarrelling and fighting over it."

'Now, this is jealousy. Now, what kind of disciples does Jesus have? As far as my observation goes, Jesus was not very fortunate in his disciples. Buddha was far more fortunate. Never in the whole life of Buddha has a disciple asked such a stupid question.

'Remember, if greed is dropped about money, immediately it will take another object, it will become focused on something else. Take responsibility, and then things start changing.

'If you take the responsibility, if you think, "I am responsible, nobody else," you will not be angry with the wife. You will not be fighting and nagging, you will not be nasty with her. You will start looking deeper and deeper. And in that very search you will become aware. That's what awareness is, that's how one becomes aware.

'And when you are fully aware of your jealousy you will be surprised, you are in for a surprise: When you are fully aware of it, it disappears. It simply disappears, not leaving even a trace behind it.

'Bring a little light inside. Meditate a little bit. Sit silently, doing nothing, looking inwards. In that stillness you will become aware of yourself and of the whole that surrounds you. That state is samadhi, and to know it is to know all, to be it is to be all.'

Transmission of the Lamp

For thousands of years India has been very fortunate to give birth to so many enlightened masters. At the same time, it has been very unfortunate in not being able to accommodate them in the country. One such master was Bodhidharma, who did not find any disciple in India and left for China. Since then, it has been asked by the seekers: Why did Bodhidharma—the greatest Zen master—go from India to China? This question has been posed repeatedly in the Zen schools of thought all over the world.

Why couldn't he find anybody in India to whom he could transmit his enlightenment?

Osho observes: 'There were scholars, pundits and philosophers available, but to them the transmission of enlightenment was not possible, as this happens only in the deepest silence, this experience can be transferred from the master to the disciple who has become so much dissolved into silence, that he even himself does not exist—it is only silence and silence alone. The scholars and pundits are not silent people—full of words, they blah blah endlessly. With them it is a psychological need, indeed a disease.

'A young man was confessing his sins to a priest, "Father, I had sex seven times last night."

The priest asked: "How many women?"

"Ah, Father, there was only one woman," answered Pat.

To which the priest said: "Well, it is not as bad as I thought. Who is the woman?"

"My wife, Father."

"Well," said the priest, "there is nothing wrong with that, son."

"I know, Father, but I just had to tell someone," replied Pat.'

Osho continues: 'There are moments when you just have to tell someone. If you don't tell, it becomes heavy on you. If you tell, you are released and relaxed. If you can find a sympathetic listener, good; otherwise just talk to yourself. But don't repress it. Repressed, it will become a burden on you. Just sit in front of the wall and have a good talk. In the beginning you will feel it a little crazy, but the more you do it, the more you will see the beauty of it. It is less violent. It does not waste somebody else's time, and it works the same way, it does the same: You are relieved. And after a good talk with the wall you will feel very, very relaxed. In fact, everybody needs to do it. The world would be better and more silent if people started talking to the walls. Try it. It will be deep meditation—knowing well that the wall is not listening. But that is not the point.

'Zen master Bodhidharma also used to sit facing the wall. After nine years of sitting he found a disciple who was worthy of the transmission of enlightenment. As they say in Hindi—*Jyoti Se Jyoti Jalaey* (light one lamp from another). Enlightenment from the master to disciple is just like the transmission of a lamp which happens in the deepest silence.'

Sense of Humour and Laughter

Osho's unique contribution to spirituality has been to incorporate celebration in it. He does not want man to renounce this life and escape to the Himalayas, but to remain in the marketplace and learn the art of meditation. Life is a unique gift that transcends religious seriousness and monotony, and enables us to expand beyond the limits of our intellect.

In his early days when he started conducting meditation camps in Mount Abu and other hill stations, Osho introduced laughter as meditation. Our chattering mind stops for a few moments when we laugh spontaneously, giving us a taste of meditation. He said, 'A sense of humour has not been recognised by any religion as a religious quality. I declare it to be the highest spiritual quality. And if we can decide that every year, at a certain appointed hour, the whole world will laugh for an hour, it will help to dispel darkness, violence and stupidity. This is because laughter is the only human characteristic which no animal possesses.'

Osho told jokes during his discourses to create an atmosphere of laughter and used it as a device to awaken people. He said, 'Laughter relaxes. And relaxation is spiritual. Laughter brings you to the earth, brings you down from your stupid ideas of being holier than thou. Laughter brings you to reality as it is. The world is a play of God, a cosmic joke. And unless you understand it as a cosmic joke you will never be able to understand the ultimate mystery. I am all for jokes, I am all for laughter.'

Osho even devised a 'laughing technique'. He said 'When you wake up in the morning, before opening your eyes, stretch like a cat. Stretch every part of your body. Enjoy the stretching, enjoy the feeling of your body becoming awake, alive. After a few minutes of stretching with your eyes still closed, laugh. For five minutes, just laugh. At first, you will just be doing it. But soon, the sound of your very attempt to laugh will cause genuine laughter. Lose yourself in it.'

George Gurdjieff: Osho's Favourite

George Gurdjieff was born near the Caucasus in Russia where still there are nomads, wandering tribes. Even sixty years of communist torture has not been able to settle those nomads, because they consider wandering to be man's birthright, and perhaps they are right. He started moving from one group to another. He learned many languages and many arts of the nomads. He learned many exercises that are not available to civilised people any more, but nomads need them.

For example; it may be very cold and the snow is falling, and to live in a tent.... Nomads know certain exercises of breathing that change the rhythm of the breath and thus the temperature of your body increases. Or if it is too hot, if you are passing through a desert, then change again to a different rhythm in order to cool down the body...your body has an automatic, inbuilt, air-conditioning system.

Gurdjieff was a master who had mysterious ways of relating to people, such that each disciple who wrote about him described him differently. Everybody who met him would carry away the image of either a good man or a rascal, and many were the arguments on this subject.

Osho called Gurdjieff a master of changing faces. He had become so efficient at this that the disciple to his right would feel one thing, while the one to his left would feel differently. With the left of his face, he would show love, and with the other, anger. And outside, one disciple would say 'What a loving man,' while the other would say, 'You are under some illusion…he was so angry!' Such mastery is beautiful. It is said no one had ever seen Gurdjieff's real face, because he was always acting. He would show you the face you needed to see; never the face that was not needed by you.

Gurdjieff enjoyed it tremendously. He did it as a reminder that we live in a fake world, where one has to keep changing faces according to the situation. It is possible to recall one's original face only through meditation. He said, 'To me, and to the Upanishads, right conduct means just the right rules of behaviour with others. You are not going to be here forever. You cannot change the world, you cannot change everybody; you can at the most change yourself. So it is better to change yourself inwardly. Don't be in a continuous fight with everybody. Faces are helpful to avoid fights, unnecessary struggle, because that dissipates energy. Preserve your energy for inner work. And that work is so significant and it needs all the energy you can give to it.'

For the outside world, remain an actor, and don't think of this as deceit. If children like toys to play with, you are not deceiving them by not giving them a real gun; let them play with the toy gun. Look at the other, at what he needs. Give out of consideration for him. This is all that is meant by right conduct.

Stop Pretending, Be Authentic

One typist was leaving her job. This was her last day in the office, and the boss was telling the old jokes that he had always been telling. Everybody was laughing, except the typist. The boss asked, 'What is the matter with you? Can't you get the jokes?'

She said, 'I got them long ago. You've been repeating them a thousand and one times, but I need not laugh anymore. Anyway tomorrow I am leaving. These fools are laughing because they have to laugh—you are the boss. So whether the joke is worth laughing at or not doesn't matter. They have to laugh, it is part of their duty. But I'm leaving, what can you do to me? I'm not laughing, you cannot make me laugh at all those rotten jokes.'

We are what we are, what we are meant to be. Yet we keep pretending to be what we are not, perhaps can never be. This is the root cause of our troubles, our suffering....

A husband may not feel loving towards his wife, but he has to please her to be comfortable at home, so he will exhibit love as a need of the moment. When he does this very often, it becomes his habit. The same is the case with wife. It happens all the time in almost all relationships. Out of compulsion, people have to pretend and show what they are not. This creates a split personality, leads to inner conflicts and one lives a life of lies. Such a life is seriously sick and lacks real happiness. How can one be happy when one is living a divided life, the external in conflict with the internal!

Osho tells a symbolic story of Hitler who was suffering from deep depression and melancholy, which psychologists said was due to a hidden inferiority complex. All the Aryan psychologists were summoned. They tried but they couldn't help; nothing emerged from their analyses. So they suggested that a Jewish psychoanalyst be called. Hitler was not ready at first to be treated by a Jew, but he had to yield since there was no way out. So, a great Jewish psychoanalyst was called. He analysed, penetrated deep into Hitler's mind, his dreams and then he suggested, 'The problem is not much. Simply repeat one thing continuously: "I am important, I am significant, I am indispensable." Let it be a mantra. Night and day, whenever you remember, repeat it: "I am important, I am significant, I am indispensable".'

Hitler said, 'Stop! You are giving me bad advice.' The psychoanalyst couldn't understand this. He said, 'What do you mean? Why do you call this bad advice?' Hitler said, 'Because whatever I say, I am such a liar I cannot believe it. If I say I am indispensable, I know it is a lie. I am saying it, but I am a liar!'

Osho explains: 'Out of lies, if you repeat something it will become a lie. Out of fear, if you do something it will become a fear again. Out of hate, if you try to love, that love will just be a hidden hate: It cannot be anything else—you are full of hate. Go to the preachers and they will say: "Try to love." they are talking nonsense because how can a person who is full of hate try to love? If he tries to love, this love will come out of hatred: It will be poisoned already, poisoned from the very source. And this is what the misery of all preachers is.'

Even the so-called teachers, educationists and moralists do not show us how to be authentic. They simply tell us to change our behaviour without going through the real transformation that takes place only through deep meditation. People become pretenders and hypocrites as they have to become what they are not. Enlightened mystics give us the science of the inner transformation and help us realise our true selves. We feel oneness of the inner and outer, the undivided self, the Advaita. For that, one need not seek psychological treatment, one should learn the Eastern way of meditation.

Be authentic and you will be in bliss!

The Inner Treasure

Existence pulsates with abundance. It embodies godliness. The Hindi word for god is *Ishwar*. The quality of godliness is *Aishwarya*. That is our inner treasure.

We carry within us an infinite treasure of spiritual wealth. There is a vast kingdom of godliness within us, immeasurable. To open this window of godliness, we need a password, and that really is 'meditation'.

We are living in the age of computers and robots. Working constantly with these mechanical gadgets, we end up behaving mechanically. And to behave like robots is not human because we do not remain masters of our lives. Some other forces of unconsciousness control us. There is no human glory or grace in such existence.

Osho reminds us: 'Bring a little more awareness to your existence. Each act has to be done less automatically than you have been doing it, and you have the key. If you are walking, don't walk like a robot. Don't keep walking as you have always walked, don't do it mechanically. Bring a little awareness to it. Slow down. Let each step be taken in full consciousness.'

'Lord Buddha used to say to his disciples that when you raise your left foot, deep down say "Left". When you raise your right foot, deep down say "Right". First say it, so you become acquainted with the process. Then slowly let the words disappear, just remember "Left, right, left, right...'"

Osho recommends: 'Try it in small acts. Eating, taking a bath, swimming, walking, talking, listening, cooking, washing your clothes.... De-automatise all processes. Remember the word: De-automatisation. That is the secret of becoming aware.

'The mind is a robot. The robot has its utility; this is the way the mind functions. You learn something; when you first learn it, you are aware. For example, if you learn to drive a car you are very alert. After all, it is so dangerous, you have to be aware. But the moment you have learned driving, this awareness is not needed. Then the robotic part of your mind takes over.' And that's when you lose consciousness.

Meditation means regaining consciousness, transcending the robotic mind. Such transcendence happens within the realm of our inner being, our consciousness. Osho says, 'Mind opens outside; meditation opens inside. Mind is a door that leads outside in the world; meditation is the door that leads you to your interiority, to the innermost shrine of your being. And suddenly, you are enlightened.'

Let Go of Anger

*Anger is an acid that can do more harm to the vessel in which it is
stored than to anything on which it is poured.*

—Mark Twain

Meditation is the way to cleanse this vessel.

A friend once asked the renowned Irish-Australian nurse
Sister Elizabeth Kenny how she managed to stay constantly cheerful.
Sister Kenny replied: 'As a girl I would often lose my temper. But
one day when I became angry with a friend over a trivial matter,
my mother gave me the sound advice that I always remember. She
said anyone who angers you actually conquers you.'

In a street in China, two persons were quarrelling and a crowd
gathered to watch. People everywhere enjoy watching such scenes.
They may be on for some serious business but when they see people
quarrelling, they forget their work and start watching. Violence has
such a great appeal. That is why all the violence, the blood and
gore on television sell like hot cakes.

Well, one of the Chinese men was rather provoked and spat
on the other person. Within minutes, the crowd of watchers had
dispersed. In China, they believe that the person who spits on the
other person first shows his weakness, because he gets provoked

in a quarrel and this means that the other has been successful in conquering you. He has aroused some poison of anger in you, compelling you to spit. And the anger ultimately hurts the person who gets angry; the receiver of the anger may not really get hurt.

One really doesn't have to be a scientist or a researcher to understand the ill-effects of anger on one's health. One has only to be sensitive. The being of an angry person starts transmitting vibrations of anger and violence around him. Just standing close to such a person may make you feel nauseated. His very presence can be uncomfortable. On the other hand, when you meditate, you feel uplifted and enveloped in a sense of comfort, of well-being.

Exhale deeply and vomit out your anger, not on others but in the emptiness around you. Deep cleanse yourself. The *Atharva Veda* says: 'Cast off anger from your heart, like an arrow from the bow, so that you may again be friends and live together absolutely in harmony.'

Osho concludes: 'Tensions are our guests, we invite them. Relaxation is our nature, we don't have to invite it. You don't have to relax, you have just to stop inviting tensions, and relaxation begins on its own. In your very core, in every fibre, in every cell of your being, relaxation percolates and assimilates. This relaxation is the beginning of meditation.'

Learn to Live and Celebrate

Remember the eternal truth: Weep and you weep alone; laugh and the whole world laughs with you.

It is your choice what you want to do with your life, how you want to live your life. You always find yourself on a crossroad and are compelled to make a choice. You could choose out of helplessness, or make a conscious choice. In helplessness, you settle for your weakness, while a conscious choice requires a certain amount of courage and self confidence—a feeling that this existence is your mother, this universe is your home. This depends on what feeling you nurture in your heart. It is not just a matter of thinking but of feeling, strong feeling.

In His discourses, Osho exhorts us to nourish our beings with positive feelings and embrace life with gratefulness and gratitude. This is the secret of the art of living—and living consciously. The art of living needs a conscious choice. It is not about drifting unconsciously in all directions. One is not as weak as one starts assuming in a state of misery. One carries within oneself a vast treasure of godliness. One has to tap into it. And the art of tapping is what meditation is all about. Then life becomes a celebration, a carnival of joys. You sing and dance and you find that the whole universe is singing and dancing with you.

'When thousands and thousands of people around the earth are celebrating, singing, dancing, ecstatic, drunk with the divine, there is no possibility of any global suicide. With such festivity and such laughter, with such sanity and health, with such naturalness and spontaneity, how can there be war?.... Life has been given to you to create, to rejoice, to celebrate. When you cry and weep, you are alone. When you celebrate, the entire existence participates with you. Only in celebration, do we meet the ultimate, the eternal. Only in celebration, do we go beyond the circle of birth and death.'

Osho tells us how to be free from pain and anguish: 'This pain is not to make you sad, remember. That's where people go amiss. This pain is just to make you more alert, because people become alert only when the arrow goes deep into their hearts and wounds them. Otherwise they don't become alert. When life is easy, comfortable, convenient, who cares? Who bothers? When a friend dies there is a possibility. When your woman leaves you alone—on those dark nights, you are lonely. You have loved that woman so much and you have staked all, and suddenly one day she is gone. Crying in your loneliness, those are the occasions when, if you use them, you can become aware. The arrow is hurting: It can be used. The pain is not to make you miserable, the pain is to make you more aware! And when you are aware, misery disappears.'

Rising Above the Din

Meditation is becoming very popular these days. People do not have the time or luxury of going to the Himalayas or to forests to meditate in isolation. They are happy meditating while living the urban life.

It was very different in the Buddha's time. He left the city and his palace as it did not give him the space to be himself. But, when he realised his potential and attained enlightenment, he returned to the city to share the learning gathered in isolation.

The city's hectic pace may compel an escape into solitude, where the meditator's individuality can blossom. But this does not mean that it can blossom only in the jungle. If we know how to, we can also meditate in the marketplace.

In a beautiful poem, Gurudev Rabindranath Tagore tells us that after enlightenment, when Gautama the Buddha returned home, his wife asked him: 'What did you attain in the jungle—was it not possible to attain it here? Why leave home, me, your child?' The Buddha remained silent.

Kabir, the mystic, lived a domestic life, worked as a weaver and yet sang: *Kabira khada bazar mein.* He not only taught meditation but preached love and asked people to gather courage, burn their houses of imagination and transform their lives. Real meditation blossoms in love, spontaneous sharing and like a flower shares its fragrance, unconditionally.

The alchemy of meditation and love transforms the ordinary love of attachment and possession into unconditional love.

Ordinary relationships are based on conditional love. It is a barter—something, in return for something. And we keep calculating the profits. This cannot bring us bliss.

Real joy comes when one shares unconditionally.

The marketplace can corrupt the minds of those who are prone to get lost in it. We need enlightened people like Kabir and Osho to show us how to rise above the world while remaining in it—just as a lotus blossoms in a pond. Delhi, with all its political tangles, cut-throat competition and mazes of ambition is a real challenge to meditate in.

Osho suggests Vipassana (watching your breath and the small gaps in the breathing)—simple meditation to be practised amidst worldly activity. When you are eating try to be attentive. Be attentive while you're walking. Don't let your activity distract your mind. Practise a dual existence of doing and being.

Doing is work (peripheral) while being is consciousness (central). As you work on the periphery, attend to the core as well.

Your activity will constitute the core. Like an actor, you can play several roles, while being rooted in consciousness. Life is just a role assigned to you by society, circumstance, culture and nation. Rejoice in it and settle in your being.

Art of Listening—*Samyak Shravan*

L istening, *shravan*, is one of the easiest and most spontaneous methods of meditation.

Osho explains this phenomenon: '*Shravan* means right listening... and this is a rare achievement. Right listening means not just fragmentary listening...I am saying something, you are listening to it...your ears are being used; but you may not be present there. If you are not present there in your totality, then it cannot be right listening....

'Right listening means you have become just your ears—your whole being is listening. No thinking inside, no thoughts, no thought process, only listening. Try it sometimes; it is a deep meditation in itself. Some birds are singing. Just become listening, forget everything—just be the ears. The wind is passing through the trees, the leaves are rustling; just become the ears, forget everything—no thought process, just listen. Become the ears. Then it is right listening, then your whole being is absorbed into it, then you are totally present.

'The Upanishads say that the esoteric, ultimate formulas of spiritual alchemy cannot be handed over to you as you are: Unconscious of yourself, with fragmentary, partial, listening. Your total being has to become receptive. They are seeds and the seeds are powerful; they will explode in you. And they will begin to grow in you, but one has to become a womb to receive them. If your ears have become wombs to receive and your total presence is there; if your whole body is listening—every fibre, every cell of the body is listening—only then these "great sentences" as they are called, the *mahavakyas*, can be delivered to you.'

You are the Masterpiece

Recently I came across a random poem aspiring to be something what it is not. It read:

> Looking to the future is something that is often done,
> What will the coming years bring except for great fun?
> How will the times change, what kind of person will I become?
> This is a question often asked; I've contemplated it some.
> To be respected, live happily, and be an example to all,
> I want to bring a smile to everyone, the big or the small.

The aspiration expressed in this poem is the aspiration that often springs in our hearts. While most of us try our best to fulfil our ambitions, often we don't succeed. Many of us feel miserable and then the failure becomes a suffering. We start finding fault with ourselves; we feel incomplete.

This constant feeling of being incomplete is the root cause of all misery. We spend our entire life trying to become something that we are not. We do all kinds of things to reach somewhere—what we assume is our goal. This goal has nothing to do with our inner reality because this goal does not originate out of our understanding of reality but from confusion and tension.

In reality, we are the seed that needs to flower. We are supposed to become what we are in our essence or potentiality. In that sense, we are perfect as we are, because we originate from the whole.

The Upanishads declare:

Om Purnamidah Purnamidam
Purnath Purnamudachyate.
Purnasya Purnamadaya
Purnamevava shisyate.

(This is the whole. That is the whole. From the whole springs the whole. Take the whole from the whole and only the whole remains.)

Meditation on this sutra can liberate us from all our anguish and misery.

This wholeness is not something that will happen in future, nor is it something to be achieved. This wholeness is pulsating within us right now, in the present moment.

The future never really comes. It is only a mental imagination functioning as conditioning. Meditation helps us become aware of this conditioning. Meditation is the key and witnessing our being without any divisions is the realisation.

In one of his discourses on Zen, Osho says: 'You are carrying a masterpiece hidden within you, but you are standing in the way. Just move aside, then the masterpiece will be revealed. Everyone is a masterpiece, because God never gives birth to anything less than that. Everyone carries that masterpiece hidden for many lives, not knowing who they are. Often, they keep trying to become someone. Drop the idea of becoming someone, because you are already a masterpiece. You cannot be improved. You have only to come to it, to know it, to realise it. God himself has created you; you cannot be improved.'

All we need to do is to settle in our witnessing consciousness

and let the flower of godliness bloom. It happens by itself. As the
Zen mystics declare:

> *Sitting silently*
> *Doing nothing*
> *The spring comes*
> *And the grass grows by itself.*

The Rigidity of Perfection

Recently I read a story: 'My name is Paul and I am a recovering perfectionist. I am also recovering from depression. The two are connected. I had been trying to do too much, too well, trying to please too many people, expecting too much of myself for too long, putting too much pressure on myself, creating too much stress. That's a lot of "too much" for one person. My self-esteem took a battering, I stopped looking forward to anything and I felt like I was useless and hopeless.' And he goes on with his story.

This is not the story of Paul alone. The world is full of such Pauls. They are going neurotic with such desires of being perfectionists and end up in the ditch of depression. What is the solution?

The wise tell us that the world is perfect as it is. You cannot ask for more. But some people are never satisfied. They want to improve things. They are so obsessed with their idea of perfection that they would improve upon God's creation too. Their obsession drives others crazy.

Here's an interesting anecdote: A king passing through a small town saw what he took to be indications of amazing marksmanship. On trees, barns and fences there were many archery boards, each with a bullet hole in the bull's eye. He could not believe his eyes. It was almost a miracle of achievement. He himself was a good marksman and had known many great marksmen in his life, but never seen anything like this. He wanted to meet the expert. He turned out to be a madman. 'This is sensational! How in the world do you do it?' he asked the madman. 'I am a good shooter too, but cannot match your skill. Please tell me!'

'Easy as pie!' said the madman, laughing uproariously. 'I shoot first and draw the circles in later!'

Osho tells us not to be perfectionists. He says that perfectionism is the root cause of all neurosis. Unless humanity gets rid of the very idea of perfection, it will never ever be sane.

The very idea of perfection has driven the whole of mankind to a state of utter madness. To think in terms of perfection means that you are thinking in terms of ideology, goals, values, shoulds, should nots...you have a certain pattern to fulfil, else you feel immensely guilty. And the pattern is bound to be such that you cannot achieve it. If you do achieve it, then it will not be of much value to your ego!

Perfectionism is a neurotic idea. An intelligent person will understand that life is an adventure, a constant exploration. That is its very joy! Perfection means a full stop. Perfection means ultimate death. There is no way to go beyond it. Perfectionists take life as a puzzle and look for solutions. But for the wise, life is a mystery to be lived with a sense of wonder.

You should be perfectly and acutely aware of the difference between a mystery and a problem. A problem is something created by the mind but a mystery is something which is already there. A problem has some ugliness in it, like a disease.

A mystery, on the other hand, is beautiful. With a problem, fights arise. Something is wrong and you have to put it right; something is missing and you must supply the missing link. With a mystery, there is no question of a fight. The moon arises in the night—that is not a problem, it is a mystery. You live with it. You dance with it. You sing with it. Or you can be silent with it. Mystery surrounds you.

Singular Devotion

There is a famous story of Sufi mystic Sheikh Farid, that a man once asked him the way to attain God. Baba Farid looked into his eyes and felt his longing. He was on his way to the river, so he asked the man to accompany him and promised to show him the way to attain God after they'd had a bath. They arrived at the river and as soon as the man plunged, Baba Farid grabbed the man's head and pushed it down into the water with great force. The man began to struggle to free himself from his grip. He was much weaker than Baba Farid but his latent strength gradually began to stir and soon it became impossible for the mystic to hold him down. The man pushed himself to the limit and was eventually able to get out of the river. He was in state of total shock while Farid was laughing loudly. After the man calmed down, Farid asked him, 'When you were under the water what desires did you have in your mind?'

He replied, 'Desires! There weren't any, there was just one desire—to get a breath of air.'

Farid said, 'This is the secret of attaining God. This is determination. And your determination awakened all your latent powers.'

In a real moment of intense determination, great strength is generated—and a man can pass from the world into truth; by determination one can awaken from the dream to the truth. In the 'Wisdom of the Sands' discourse, Osho shares this insight: 'It is only through intensity that one arrives. When all your desires, all your passions become one flame, it is intensity. When there is only one desire left inside you and your total being supports that one, it is intensity. It is exactly what the word says: In-tensity. The opposite word is ex-tensity. You are spread out, you have a thousand and one desires, many fragmentary desires—one going to the north, one going to the south. You are being pulled apart. You are not one, you are a crowd. And if you are a crowd you will be miserable. If you are a crowd you will never feel any fulfilment. You don't have any centre. Intensity means creating a centre in yourself. When all the arrows are coming towards the centre, when all the fragments are joined together, integration arises. Becoming centred, concentrated inwards, that is the meaning of intensity. In moments of danger when all your thoughts disappear, the crowd will become one. In that moment you will be one single individual, indivisible. You will be an undivided, single unity. Facing death has generated an intensity. Even love can evoke a similar intensity. All else becomes irrelevant, peripheral. When such intensity arises in meditation, it brings you to the ultimate. You arrive home.'

Merge to Re-emerge

A mother hugs her child. A friend holds the hand of her friend or hugs her. A child comes running into the father's arms when he returns from work. All these acts involve touch to form a connection and transferring one's energy to the other.

The street dogs play amongst themselves, jumping and wrestling with each other. This gives them energy. Potted plants and trees rooted in the earth lean towards each other in order to derive energy from each other. The sun rises early in the morning giving energy to chirping birds and trees. People who are fortunate enough to listen to the early song of birds are also rejuvenated likewise.

Our universe is one big family supporting life in all its forms with energy. While scientists term it energy, mystics deem it to be a universal satsang, a divine communion. The mystics have known this communion for eternity and remind us about its presence in a variety of expressions.

It is heartening to know that even scientists are waking up to this phenomenon; they have started engaging in experiments which prove the spiritual revelations of the sages—*kan kan me bhagwan* i.e. every atom is divine. We are composed of these atoms. But scientists call it bioenergy.

By sharing energy, we exercise a healing effect on one another.

This makes us realise that we are interdependent at many levels—from plants to birds to people. This is the realisation of a meditator.

Recently, a biological research team at Bielefeld University in Germany made a groundbreaking discovery, showing that plants can draw an alternative source of energy from other plants. Members of professor Dr Olaf Kruse's biological research team confirmed, for the first time, that the green algae *Chlamydomonas reinhardtii* not only engages in photosynthesis, but also draws energy from other plants. Many psychologists have also started working on the energy phenomenon. Some of them feel that just like flowers, humans too need water and light to grow. Our physical bodies are like sponges, soaking up the environment.

The psychologist Ms. Bader-Lee suggests that the field of bioenergy is now ever-evolving and that studies on the plant and animal world will soon translate and demonstrate an energy that metaphysicians have known all along—that humans can heal each other simply through energy transfer just as plants do. Humans can absorb and heal through other humans, animals and any part of nature. That's why being around nature is often uplifting and energising for all of us.

The scientific community approaches every manifestation of nature from outside while sages and yogis undertake an inner journey. In this way, they are connected to everything that surrounds them, from within. It is a conscious approach that operates only from consciousness to consciousness. And it is not merely a matter of concentration—it is all-inclusive.

Osho concludes that matter and consciousness are not two separate things. What we call matter is consciousness asleep and what we know as consciousness is matter awakened. They are different manifestations of the same thing. Existence is 'one' and that 'one' is godliness or Brahman. When that 'one' is asleep it appears as matter and when awake it is consciousness. So matter and consciousness are only utilitarian terms. They are not really different.

The Sutra of Breathing

Whether it is Tantra or Yoga or Tao, all these ancient spiritual streams emphasise on one thing and that is to be in tune with the breath if we have to embark on an inner journey and its deeper realms of consciousness. In *Vigyan Bhairav Tantra*, Devi Parvati asks: 'O Shiva, what is your reality? What is this wonder-filled universe? What constitutes seed? Who centres the universal wheel? What is this life beyond form pervading forms? How may we enter it fully, above space and time, names and descriptions?'

Shiva replies: 'Radiant One, this experience may dawn between two breaths. After breath comes in (down) and just before turning up (out)—the beneficence.' Thus, Lord Shiva gives some powerful methods of breathing to start with. He tells her that this way, one can experience the fundamental nature of this universe and can go beyond the space and time to understand this transcendental truth. And after this he gives three more techniques of breathing in answer to her questions.

The meditation on breath differs when you are following a certain path, such as Yoga, Vipassana or Tao, but the thread, the sutra of breathing, remains the same. The breath plays a pivotal role in the transformation of a seeker and his expansion of consciousness. Gautama, the Buddha said: 'Be aware of your breath as it is coming in, going out—coming in, going out. Be aware. When the breath is going in move with it, and when the breath is going out move with it. Do simply this: Going in, going out, with the breath.'

This one technique has worked wonders for millions of people in the Asian countries. The whole of Asia tried and lived with this technique for centuries. Thousands of seekers attained self-realisation through this single technique. People experience immense peace and wonderful spaces during their practice.

What is the secret? Osho explains: 'Your breath is a bridge between you and your body. Constantly, breath is bridging you to your body, connecting you, relating you to your body. Not only is the breath a bridge to your body, it is also a bridge between you and the universe. The body is just the universe which has come to you, which is nearer to you. Your body is part of the universe. Everything in the body is part of the universe. It is the nearest approach to the universe.'

Breath is the bridge. If the bridge is broken, you are no more in the universe. You move into some unknown dimension; then you cannot be found in space and time. So thirdly, breath is also the bridge between you, and space and time. One has to ride on the phenomenon of breath with full awareness. As Osho points out breath has two points:

'One is where it touches the body and the universe, and another is where it touches you and that which transcends the universe. We know only one part of the breath, when it moves into the universe, into the body as we know it. But it is always moving from the body to the "no-body," from the "no-body" to the body. We do not know the other point. If you become aware of the other point, the other part of the bridge, the other pole of the bridge, you will be transformed and transplanted into a different dimension.'

The Escape Within

The series of earthquakes in Nepal and India shook the world deeply and scientists in the West are expecting more earthquakes to shake the planet. Professor Bill McGuire of the University College London was quoted in *Newsweek* as saying, 'There are geological systems all around the planet with unstable volcanoes that are susceptible: When it comes to risk, I'm afraid there is a very, very long list.'

The insensitivity of our lifestyle towards the Earth has done tremendous harm. While scientists and politicians are busy providing solutions to disaster situations, here's the story Osho told about a Japanese Zen master who was invited to a satsang at a mansion.

'A few seekers had gathered for the session. As the master started talking, there was an earthquake. Japan experiences earthquakes on a frequent basis. They were all assembled on the seventh floor of a seven-storey building. Everybody tried to escape. The host, running by, stopped to see what had happened to the Zen master. The master was there with not even a ripple of anxiety on his face. He sat with his eyes closed, just as he was before the tremors began.

Seeing this, the host felt a little guilty. The other guests had already gone downstairs, but he stopped. Though trembling with fear, he sat down beside the master. After the earthquake was over, the disciples began to tiptoe back to where the master was sitting in silence. When they asked him why he did not run away, he replied, "I also escaped, but you escaped outwardly, I escaped within. Your escape is useless because wherever you are going there is an earthquake, so it is meaningless, it makes no sense. You may reach the sixth storey or the fifth or the fourth, but there too is an earthquake. I escaped to a point within me where no earthquake ever reaches, cannot reach. I entered my centre.'"

Thus, Osho concludes that meditation brings you face to face with reality. Once you know what life is, you never bother about death. Meditation is the only way to discover 'deathlessness'.

Mirdad

The maverick mystic Mirdad reveals the real mystery of prayer, which is the fragrance of heart that has been purified by the cleansing process of meditation or some alternate spiritual practice. Without deep meditation, our prayer becomes the by-product of our conditioning. Then it's merely the prayer of Hindu or Muslim conditioning. The real prayer is beyond all this conditioning.

Osho explains that you need not go to the temple to pray, but wherever you pray, you create a temple, an invisible temple. Wherever somebody bows down in prayer to existence, that becomes sacred. To a praying heart, any stone becomes Kaaba, any water becomes Ganga water. To a praying heart, each tree is a Bodhi Tree. There is nothing official about prayer. There exists no law about prayer. It is a love-affair between a human heart and the Existence or Life.

Life itself is the unofficial temple of prayer.

Leo Tolstoy has written a beautiful story: 'Three men became very famous saints in Russia.

'The highest priest of the country was very much disturbed—obviously, because people were not coming to him, people were going to those three saints, and he had not even heard their names. And how could they be saints?—In Christianity a saint is a saint only when the church recognises him as a saint. The English word "saint" comes from "sanction"; when the church sanctions somebody as a saint, then he is a saint. What nonsense! That a saint has to be certified by the church, by the organised religion, by the priests—as if it has nothing to do with inner growth but some outer recognition; as if it is a title given by a government, or a degree, an honorary degree, conferred by a university.

'The high priest was certainly very angry. He took a boat because those three saints used to live on the far side of a lake. He went in the boat. Those three saints were sitting under a tree. They were very simple people, peasants, uneducated. They touched the feet of the highest priest, and the priest was very happy. He thought, "Now I will put them right—these are not very dangerous people. I was thinking they would be rebels or something." He asked them, "How did you become saints?"

'They said, "We don't know! We don't know that we are saints either. People have started calling us saints and we go on trying to convince them that we are not, we are very simple people, but they don't listen. The more we argue that we are not, the more they worship us! And we are not very good at arguing either."

'The priest was very happy. He said, "What is your prayer? Do you know how to pray?"

'They looked at each other. The first said to the second, "You say." The second said to the third, "You say, please."

'The priest said, "Say what your prayer is! Are you saying Our Lord's Prayer or not?"

'They said, "To be frank with you, we don't know any prayer. We have invented a prayer of our own and we are very embarrassed— how to say it? But if you ask we have to say it. We have heard that God is a trinity: The Father, the Son and the Holy Ghost. We are three and he is also three, so we have made a small prayer of our own: 'You are three, we are three: Have mercy on us!'"

'The priest said, "What nonsense! Is this prayer? You fools, I will teach you the right prayer." And he recited The Lord's Prayer.

'And those three poor people said, "Please repeat it once more, because we are uneducated, we may forget."

'He repeated it and they asked, "Once more—we are three, repeat it at least three times." So he repeated it again, and then very happy, satisfied, he went back in his boat.

'Just in the middle of the lake he was surprised, his boatman was surprised: Those three poor people were coming running on the water! And they said, "Wait! Please one more time—we have forgotten the prayer!"

'Now it was the turn of the priest to touch their feet, and he said, "Forget what I have said to you. Your prayer has been heard, my prayer has not been heard yet. You continue as you are continuing. I was utterly wrong to say anything to you. Forgive me!"'

Prayer is a state of simplicity. It is not of words but of silence.

—As told by Osho in his discourse 'Be Still and Know'

The Silence of the Words:
The Book of Mirdad

New books are being published every day, and millions of books are available worldwide. Still, many old books continue to remain popular because people just love reading them. The thirst for knowledge and wisdom, fiction and fun is insatiable. Once in a while we come across a book that transforms us and changes the course of our life.

Osho loved reading books and he did read more than 100,000 books, which are now part of his personal library. Osho makes a special mention of one unique book which not many people know of. He says: 'There are millions of books in the world, but *The Book of Mirdad* stands out far above any other book in existence. It is unfortunate that very few people are acquainted with this book because it is not a religious scripture. It is a parable, a fiction, but containing oceanic truth. It is a small book, but the man who gave birth to this book—and mind my words, I am not saying "the man who wrote this book", nobody wrote this book—was an unknown, a nobody. And because he was not a novelist, he never wrote again; just that single book contains his whole experience. The name of the man was Mikhail Naimy.

'It is an extraordinary book in the sense that you can read it and miss it completely, because the meaning of the book is not in the words of the book. The meaning of the book is running side by side in silence between the words, between the lines, in the gaps. If you are in a state of meditativeness—if you are not only reading a fiction but you are encountering the whole religious experience of a great human being, absorbing it; not intellectually understanding but existentially drinking it—the words are there but they become secondary. Something else becomes primary: The silence that those words create, the music that those words create. The words affect your mind, and the music goes directly to your heart.

Reading a book like *The Book of Mirdad* is an art by itself. Osho tells us: 'And it is a book to be read by the heart, not by the mind. It is a book not to be understood, but experienced. It is something phenomenal. Millions of people have tried to write books so that they can express the inexpressible, but they have utterly failed. I know only one book, *The Book of Mirdad*, which has not failed; and if you cannot get to the very essence of it, it will be your failure, not the author's. He has created a perfect device of words, parables, situations. If you allow it, the book becomes alive and something starts happening to your being.'

Mikhail Naimy writes: 'You are the tree of life. Beware of fractioning yourselves. Set not a fruit against a fruit, a leaf against a leaf, a bough against a bough; nor set the stem against the roots; nor set the tree against the mother-soil. That is precisely what you do, when you love one part more than the rest or to the exclusion of the rest.'

Our life functions in an organic connectivity. We are one life—and this life itself is godliness. While we are creating conflict constantly, living in man-made divisions of religions, races and nations, a man of meditation comes to realise that there exist no divisions and fractions in life. All divisions exist only in the overdeveloped heads and underdeveloped hearts of people. We are conscious of the leaves, branches and stems of the tree, but we cannot see the roots of the tree, the source of one life. This is the real misery of men on earth.

'No love is love that subjugates the lover. No love is love that draws a woman to a man only to breed more women and men and thus perpetuate their bondage to the flesh,' writes Naimy.

Those who can see neither before nor after believe this segment of eternity to be itself eternity. They cling to the delusion of duality... not knowing that the rule of life is Unity.

Hugs for Emotional Nourishment

After hugging millions of people around the world, Mata Amritanandamayi embraced another headline-making project. She contributed a whopping ₹100 crore for cleaning the river Ganga, under Prime Minister Modi's pet project, the Swachch Bharat Abhiyaan.

Amma travels the world offering hugs and a message of unconditional love. Hug someone you love today. Hugs could give your heart an emotional nourishment. Several books have been written on the benefits of hugging. In recent times, this human practice called hugging has evolved into a therapy. Marcia, a well-known hug therapist recommends four hugs a day for survival, eight hugs a day for maintenance and twelve hugs a day for growth.

Life does not believe in such arithmetic, though it is probably true that every human being needs certain amount of touch and certain number of hugs. The child may need more hugs than a grown-up. But then, not everybody grows up with the same speed, so in some cases a seemingly grown-up person may need more hugs than a child.

Our society does not recognise this human need and its response to this need is hardly sympathetic. No wonder then that it continues to suffer. People are not open to this human emotion though privately everyone loves to love and be loved in return. So the hugs have become very limited to only between close relationships. There may be some lukewarm hugging between friends, which is not very nourishing. One needs more than that. What is then the alternative? Hug a tree! It won't get you into any trouble. And make it into a meditation.

Hugging a tree is an ancient technique of meditation that can be found in the *Vigyana Bhairav Tantra*, one of the oldest meditation manuals in existence, and composed in Sanskrit. Here is what Osho says on the subject of hugging a tree for meditation. 'Leave one hour aside every day for a prayerful state of mind, and don't make your prayer a verbal affair. Make it a feeling thing. Rather than talking with the head, feel it. Go and touch the tree, hug the tree, kiss the tree; close your eyes and be with the tree as if you are with your beloved. Feel it. And soon you will come to a deep understanding of what it means to put the self aside, of what it means to become the other. Only once in a while it will happen—because it has to happen in spite of you, that's why only once in a while.' Yes and women can do it just as well as men.

'Have you ever said hello to a tree? Try it, and one day you will be surprised: The tree also says hello in her tongue, in her own language. Hug a tree, and a day will come soon when you will feel that it was not only you who were hugging the tree—the tree was responding, you were also hugged by the tree, although the tree has no hands. But it has its own way of expressing its joy, its sadness, its anger, its fear.'

Hug a tree and relax into it. Feel its green shape rushing into your being.

In Tune with Nature

There is a beautiful story about Saint Francis who had a really unique way of praying to god.

Once he and his companions were making a trip through the Spoleto Valley near the town of Bevagna. Suddenly, Francis spotted a great number of birds of all varieties. There were doves, crows and all sorts of birds. Swept up in the moment, Francis left his friends on the road and ran after the birds, who patiently waited for him. He greeted them in his usual way, expecting them to scurry off into the air as he spoke. But they moved not. Filled with awe, he asked them if they would stay awhile and listen to the Word of God. He said to them: 'My brother and sister birds, you should praise your Creator and always love him: He gave you feathers for clothes, wings to fly and all other things that you need. It is God who made you noble among all creatures, making your home in thin, pure air. Without sowing or reaping, you receive God's guidance and protection.'

At this the birds began to spread their wings, stretch their necks and gaze at Francis, rejoicing and praising God in a wonderful way according to their nature. Francis then walked right through the middle of them, turned around and came back, touching their heads and bodies with his tunic.

Saint Francis used to talk to trees. He would say to an almond tree, 'Sister, sing to me of God!' He would go to the river and talk to it and the fishes that were in the flowing waters. Nothing in existence was a stranger to him. The trees, the fish and the river do not understand our language, but they did understand what Saint Francis spoke to them. The language of love can be understood in silence by the inanimate objects. Even these come to life with the touch of love.

Man has forgotten to relate or communicate genially to his fellow men. Then how will he communicate with trees and rocks, the fishes and the rivers, the whole nature in all its splendour? The whole idea of ecology depends on man's ability to communicate with nature. For long, all his training and education has taught him to dominate, exploit and destroy the nature. Communication with nature has not been his education.

Here meditation can play a vital role. As a first step, meditation creates a space in which man learns to relate with himself, with his own inner nature. Remember, I am talking about relating with and not conquering and controlling the inner nature. One can relate only in friendliness.

Then comes the next step of relating with nature outside—the trees, the mountains, the rivers and the whole cosmos. The outer ecology ultimately depends on the inner ecology of the man. If a man is loving and sensitive, his love and sensitivity will radiate to the trees, animals, birds, fellow human beings and the whole earth. His inner level of growth will determine his relationship with the outside world.

Meditation essentially changes the inner climate of man, brings harmony to his being and creates a balance in his inner ecology. Once we become friendly with our own being, we become sensitive and compassionate with others too. A natural reverence flows through all our relations.

Talking on Khalil Gibran's Messiah, Osho says, 'I will say religion is reverence for life. And if you don't have reverence for life, you cannot conceive the whole of existence—the trees, and the birds and the animals—as different expressions of the same energy. In the source we are brothers and sisters with the animals and the birds and the trees; and if you start feeling this brotherhood, this sisterhood, you will find the first taste of what religion is.'

We celebrate the World Environment Day every year. It will be a good step to first take care of our inner environment so that the same positive energy in turn flows outwards to the outer ecology. The outer ecology is being destroyed because the inner nature has been destroyed. It is just an outcome.

Osho says: 'When man is no more whole inside—divided, in conflict, like a fighting mob, in a crowd—that man creates disturbance in nature also. And these are related. When nature is destroyed and the natural systems are destroyed, then man is more destroyed. Then again nature goes on affecting man and man goes on affecting nature. It is a vicious circle.'

SELF

IN

SILENCE

Self in Silence

There is an Arabian proverb: When you have spoken the word, it reigns over you. When it is unspoken you reign over it.

Words are very important tools of communication. Words delight us when they are used by intelligent people with full awareness and words bring calamities when they are used without awareness. Speech without awareness can be a dangerous weapon as it can harm people far and wide. That's why the enlightened masters such as the Buddha advised his disciples about right speech, saying that if we cannot perform right speech, we had better not speak, as it is said, 'Silence is golden'.

It is certainly true that right speech brings happiness, harmony and wisdom to life. On the contrary, wrong speech brings conflict, division, confusion and suffering to life. The poet Robert Frost observed: 'Half the world is composed of people who have something to say and can't, and the other half who have nothing to say and keep on saying it'. This situation creates a huge conflict between the two halves. Those who have nothing to say have always been clamouring for the freedom to say it, as they think it is their birthright. And everybody in the modern world is fighting for his birthright. With such endless fights about the birthright, the right expression gets lost in all kinds of noises between my right and your right, and the fights continue to erupt on regular basis.

Jesus Christ warned humanity: 'But I tell you that men will have to give account on the day of judgement for every careless word they have spoken. For by your words you will be acquitted, and by your words you will be condemned.'

Osho says: 'Ordinarily we understand only words. We are prepared to understand only words, not silence. We are educated to understand language and all its complexities. Nobody helps us to go beyond language, to go beyond words, to reach the wordless space within us.

'Silence is the explosion of intelligence. Silence means: You are just uncluttered spaciousness. It means you have put aside the whole furniture of the mind—the thoughts, the desires, the memories, the fantasies, the dreams, you have pushed them all aside. You are just looking into existence directly. That is silence. And to be in tune with existence even for a single moment is enough to make you aware of things. One is that you are eternal. Once you realise this, fear disappears. And the society exists through exploiting your fear; hence, it teaches you from the school to the university, it devotes almost one-third of your life in learning words, language and logic. It is not concerned at all that you should understand silence.

'That's the function of a Master: To undo all that the society has done to you, to help you to go beyond words. And you can experience it happening here—you can hear the silence. And when you hear it, there is immediate understanding. Understanding comes like a shadow following silence.'

Osho concludes: 'To understand words and to hear words is very simple. Anybody can do it; just a little education about language is needed, nothing much. But a tremendous transformation is needed to hear silence and to understand silence…. Silence is the basic requirement of understanding God, the basic requirement to know truth.... Silence can be profane too. Silence can be sacred too. Silence has as many nuances, as many dimensions as your being has. It is multidimensional.'

Just Be Natural

There's an ancient story, from the time of Confucius and Lao Tzu. Both were contemporaries. Confucius was younger than Lao Tzu but more popular as a philosopher. His thoughts influenced China in a very big way then, and to this day his philosophy of life continues to dominate the Chinese mentality. Lao Tzu was a mystic, like an Upanishadic sage of India, who had a transcendental wisdom of self-realisation. He had nothing to do with any philosophy, social morality or code of conduct. He was a simple man with profound understanding of life. But he could not influence people as much as Confucius could. He never bothered.

It has been reported that Confucius went to see Lao Tzu and asked, 'What do you say about morality? What do you say about how to cultivate good character?' Lao Tzu laughed loudly and said, 'If you are immoral, only then does the question of morality arise. And if you don't have any character, only then you think about character. A man of character is absolutely oblivious of the fact that anything like character exists. A man of morality does not know what the word "moral" means. So don't be foolish! And don't try to cultivate it. Just be natural.'

Osho loves Lao Tzu: 'And this man (Lao Tzu) had such tremendous energy that Confucius started trembling. He couldn't stand him. He escaped. He became afraid—as one becomes afraid near an abyss. When he came back to his disciples, who were waiting outside under a tree, the disciples could not believe it. This man had been going to emperors, the greatest emperors, and they had never seen any nervousness in him. And he was trembling, and cold perspiration was coming, pouring out from all over his body. They couldn't believe it—what had happened? What had this man Lao Tzu done to their teacher? They asked him and he said, "Wait a little. Let me collect myself. This man is dangerous."'

There is another significant Taoist story of that time: 'An old follower of Lao Tzu, who was ninety-years old, was busy pulling water from the well, together with his young son. Confucius happened to pass by. He saw the old man and his young son yoked together, pulling water from the well. He was filled with compassion. He went up to the old man and said: "Do you not know, you foolish fellow, that now we harness horses or oxen to do this job? Why are you unnecessarily tiring yourself and this young boy?"

'The old man said, "Hush! Pray speak softly lest my son hears! Come after some time when my boy goes for lunch." Confucius was perplexed. When the youth left, he asked the old man, "Why would you not let your son hear what I said?" He replied, "I am ninety-years old and yet I have the strength to work side by side with a youth of thirty. If I engage horses to pull the water, my son will not have the same strength at ninety that I have now. So I pray to you, do not talk of this before my son. It is a question of his health. We have heard that in towns horses pull water from the well. We also know that there are machines that do this job as well. But then, what will my son do? What will happen to his health, his constitution?"'

Osho concludes: 'Work and rest are interdependent. For example: We want to sleep soundly. He who wishes to sleep soundly needs to work hard. He who does not toil, cannot sleep soundly. Lao Tzu says, "Work and rest are both united. If you wish to relax, toil hard."'

'Strive so hard that relaxation falls on you. Now if we think the Aristotelian way, work and rest are different and opposite. If I am fond of rest and comfort, and wish to sleep soundly, I shall just sit around the whole day and do nothing. But he who rests in the day, destroys his repose of the night. Rest has to be earned through labour. Or else you shall have to pass a restless night.

'Confucius' way of thinking is Aristotelian, therefore the West honoured Confucius very much these last 300 years. It is only now that Lao Tzu is rising in their esteem.'

The Feminine Mystery and Its Power

Whenever some important visionary wants to bring out any change or transformation of India, he leads the country men with the slogan *Bharat mata ki jai*, or *Vandemataram* (Glory to Mother India or long live the motherland). People often wonder: Does such an entity as Bharat mata exist? Because we have never seen her!

There is no such entity anywhere in India in physical form. It exists in the collective psyche of the country's men and women. That's why the invoking works—and works wonders. That's the inner secret of the eternal India—the imperishable India. India remains united under the influence of mysterious feminine power and it is in turmoil whenever it goes astray.

Osho contemplates: 'Whether it is the birth of matter or whether it is the birth of consciousness; whether the earth is born or heaven, everything is born through the mystery that lies hidden in the depths of Existence. Therefore I have said that those who have looked upon God as mother—as Durga or Amba—their understanding is much deeper than those who look upon Him as Father. If God exists anywhere, He is feminine, for man does not have the ability and the patience to give birth to such a vast Universe. That which gives birth to the myriads of stars and moons must have a womb, without which it is impossible.'

He adds: 'Have you ever seen the image of Kali? She is the mother, She is terrible! In one hand she holds a human skull! She is the mother—Her eyes are filled with the ocean of tenderness. Down below—She stands on the chest of someone! Someone lies crushed under Her feet! Why? Because that which creates, destroys also. Destruction is the other part of creation. Those were wonderful people who conceived this image. They were people with great imagination who could visualise great possibilities.'

The words of the Chinese mystic Lao Tzu are conclusive:

The Tao is called the Great Mother
empty yet inexhaustible,
it gives birth to infinite worlds.

There's No Shortcut

The recent issue of *The New York Times*, in one of its articles, tells us that meditation is exploding in popularity. There are classes to learn meditation in all its forms: Mindfulness-based stress reduction, Transcendental Meditation, Zen and more. There are meditation events with power-networking opportunities built in. Drop by the Port Authority Trans-Hudson (commonly called PATH) in New York, and you can mingle with people in tech, film, fashion and the arts. Pay a visit to the World Economic Forum in Davos, Switzerland, and you get to do an early morning guided meditation with global leaders. As the editor-in-chief of *The Huffington Post* Arianna Huffington said, 'CEOs are increasingly coming out of the closet as meditators.'

Another newspaper reported that researchers mapping the brain activity of Tango dancers suggest that Tango has the capacity to transport a person to the same mental state as people who meditate. One experiment, presented by the US National Library of Medicine, established that Argentine Tango could be as effective as mindful meditation in reducing symptoms of stress, anxiety and depression.

The notion about the effect of meditation that it reduces stress, anxiety and depression has become prevalent all over the world. And it is a fact. It does. But in ancient time, this was not the original purpose of meditation. When the ancient sages were practising meditation, they were not thinking of freedom from stress or anxiety. They were meditating to attain self-realisation or illumination. It was self-enquiry or self-actualisation. Now meditation is being sold on a very large scale to the corporate world by most of the modern gurus with temptations, with certain packages of decision-making, increasing the productivity of the workers in the factories, etc. The power of meditation is being exploited for mundane achievements.

People are being misled on a very large scale. For example, Patanjali yoga has been reduced to mere physical asanas for better health and nothing further or deeper and the same is being done to meditation. All kinds of new methods are being invented and promoted as the short-cut to happiness and ultimately the enlightenment by those who want to turn into a big business, comparable to yoga. These teachers are mostly flourishing in the West as well as in the Eastern countries such as India and Japan, the sacred home to Vipassana and Zen. The mystic saint Kabir had warned about such teachers: 'Andha andham thelia dono koop padant (The blind led the blind and both have fallen into the well)'.

Describing this situation, Osho says: 'The ordinary man is living a very abnormal life, because his values are upside down. Money is more important than meditation; logic is more important than love; mind is more important than heart; power over others is more important than power over one's own being. Mundane things are more important than finding some treasures which death cannot destroy.'

Meditators's Mark

Gautam Buddha, Tirthankar Mahavira and many other awakened ones have preached reverence for all life forms. This includes sensitivity towards and abstinence from killing of animals for our pleasure.

Osho tells us: 'It seems to me that killing animals for eating is not very far away from killing human beings. They differ only in their body, in their shape, but it is the same life that you are destroying. With new technology, the earth is perfectly capable of giving you food. You can make it as tasteful as you want and you can give it any flavour. Destroying life for the sake of taste is disgusting. In destroying life you are destroying many qualities within yourself. In this way you cannot become a Buddha. You cannot have that purity of consciousness, that sensitivity.'

A meditator who does sadhana is supposed to be conscious in every moment, as life presents problems at each step. Osho explains this with a story: 'The Buddha had told his bhikkhus, "Whatsoever is given to you when you go begging, never reject it. That is insulting." And he was careful, because if he allowed people to reject anything then they would choose good things only. "So accept whatever is given gracefully, thankfully, and eat it. And don't throw away anything."

'One day, a bird dropped a piece of meat in a monk's begging bowl. The monk was in a bind as he could neither empty the contents of his begging bowl nor eat the meat as both would amount to flouting the Buddha's order. So he came into the commune and asked the Buddha what to do.

'Even Gautam Buddha, for a moment, was in a dilemma. If he said, "Throw it away," then he would allow an exception which would soon become a rule. If he said, "Eat it," then he is allowing meat to be eaten. But then he thought, birds are not going to drop meat every day. So he said, "We are vegetarians, and we will remain as such, but you I allow to eat this meat, so that nobody ever throws out anything which is given to him." But Buddhists took this to be an assent in support of non-vegetarianism. So Buddhists in China, Japan and Korea—the whole of Asia, except India, eat meat.

'A meditator cannot allow himself such leeway if he seeks enlightenment. To attain Buddha's nature one must remain true to the teachings of the Buddha, instead of quoting an idle statement to indulge one's appetites.'